Airway Epithelium

Colloquium Series on Integrated Systems Physiology: From Molecule to Function to Disease

Editors

D. Neil Granger, *Louisiana State University Health Sciences Center–Shreveport*
Joey P. Granger, *University of Mississippi Medical Center*

Physiology is a scientific discipline devoted to understanding the functions of the body. It addresses function at multiple levels, including molecular, cellular, organ, and system. An appreciation of the processes that occur at each level is necessary to understand function in health and the dysfunction associated with disease. Homeostasis and integration are fundamental principles of physiology that account for the relative constancy of organ processes and bodily function even in the face of substantial environmental changes. This constancy results from integrative, cooperative interactions of chemical and electrical signaling processes within and between cells, organs, and systems. This eBook series on the broad field of physiology covers the major organ systems from an integrative perspective that addresses the molecular and cellular processes that contribute to homeostasis. Material on pathophysiology is also included throughout the eBooks. The state-of the-art treatises were produced by leading experts in the field of physiology. Each eBook includes stand-alone information and is intended to be of value to students, scientists, and clinicians in the biomedical sciences. Since physiological concepts are an ever-changing work-in-progress, each contributor will have the opportunity to make periodic updates of the covered material.

Published titles

(for future titles please see the Web site, www.morganclaypool.com/page/lifesci)

Airway Epithelium
Jonathan Widdicombe
www.morganclaypool.com

ISBN: 9781615043743   paperback

ISBN: 9781615043750   ebook

DOI: 10.4199/C00063ED1V01Y201206ISP036

A Publication in the Morgan & Claypool Publishers Life Sciences series

COLLOQUIUM SERIES ON INTEGRATED SYSTEMS PHYSIOLOGY: FROM MOLECULE TO FUNCTION TO DISEASE

Lecture #36

Series Editors: D. Neil Granger, LSU Health Sciences Center, and Joey P. Granger, University of Mississippi Medical Center

Series ISSN
ISSN 2154-560X   print
ISSN 2154-5626   electronic

Airway Epithelium

Jonathan Widdicombe
Professor
Department of Physiology and Membrane Biology
University of California-Davis School of Medicine

COLLOQUIUM SERIES ON INTEGRATED SYSTEMS PHYSIOLOGY:
FROM MOLECULE TO FUNCTION TO DISEASE #36

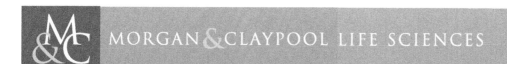

MORGAN & CLAYPOOL LIFE SCIENCES

ABSTRACT

The airways are lined with a film of fluid ~10 μm deep that acts as the first line of defense against inhaled pathogens, dirt, and noxious vapors. Transepithelial fluid movements driven by active transepithelial ion transport serve to regulate the depth of this "airway surface liquid". In the larger airways, a mucus gel derived from both glands and surface epithelium entraps inhaled particles, which are then removed by the coordinated beating of cilia. Both glands and epithelium secrete a wide variety of antimicrobial and other protective substances in addition to mucins. Substances released across the basolateral surface of the epithelium attract leukocytes and influence neighboring tissues. Here, after reviewing the basic structure of mammalian airway epithelium, I discuss its various defensive functions and how they are altered in airway disease.

KEYWORDS

airway epithelium, mucus secretion, antimicrobials, active ion transport, transepithelial fluid movement, submucosal glands, mucociliary clearance, cystic fibrosis, asthma.

Contents

CHAPTER 1

Overview

The luminal surface of mammalian airways is lined with a continuous sheet of ciliated epithelium, which in the largest airways penetrates the submucosa in the form of exocrine glands. Surface and gland epithelia act as barriers, perform vectorial transport of ions and water, and secrete mucus and a wide variety of other substances. By so doing they influence the depth and composition of a film of liquid on the luminal aspect of the epithelium, the so-called airway surface liquid (ASL). ASL is continuous; at no point is there contact between the epithelial cells and the air. Thus, all inhaled particles and noxious gases first encounter the ASL, which is central to the defense of the lung. In health, the ASL is ~10 μm deep, corresponding to ~1 μl of liquid per cm^2 of mucosal surface. It consists of two layers. A mucus gel, of variable thickness, lies on the tips of the cilia. The cilia themselves are bathed in a gel-free sol that is almost invariably the same depth as their length (i.e., ~5 μm) (Figure 1). The cilia beat in a coordinated fashion within the sol, and their tips contact the underside of the gel and propel it towards the mouth and out of the airways at ~4 mm/min [1].

The separation of sol and gel may reflect the inability of cilia to penetrate the gel; the effective pore radius of mucous gels is ~100 nm [5], whereas cilia are 200 nm in diameter. Also, electron micrographs show a dense layer at the base of the gel (Figure 1B and C) that may well have a pore size much less than that of the main body of the gel. Finally, penetration of the gel between the cilia will be hindered by their close spacing (200 nm between adjacent outer surfaces) and by their dense glycocalyx [6].

There is a progressive decrease in the depth of the mucus blanket with increasing airway generation. In health, in the largest human airways, it is generally about ~5 μm deep, but is no longer easily recognizable after about generation 15 [7]. The primary function of the mucous gel is to entrap large inhaled particles, and the decline in gel thickness distally reflects the patterns of large particle deposition (see following). Smaller particles, depositing in airways beyond the mucous gel, are removed predominantly by phagocytosis performed by airway macrophages, other leukocytes, and the epithelium itself [8]. In the latter case, the particles are frequently transcytosed and ultimately disposed of by phagocytes in the lymph system or interstitium [9]. However, the proportion of particles cleared by this transepithelial route is unknown.

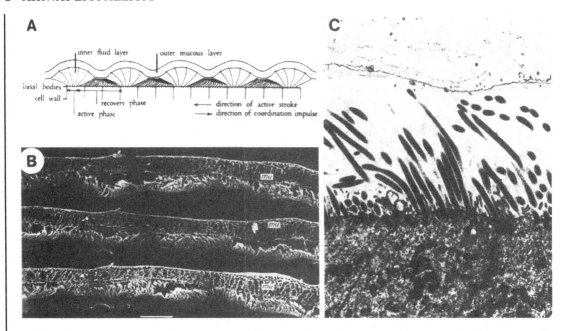

FIGURE 1: The two layers of the airway surface liquid: Periciliary sol and mucous gel. A) As originally described by Lucas & Douglas [2]. B) In rapidly frozen specimens of cultures of rabbit tracheal epithelium [3]. mu = mucous blanket. Scale bar = 10 μm. C) In rat tracheal epithelium [4].

What is the pattern of large particle deposition? In rural areas, a liter of air contains approximately 5×10^6 particles, a number that increases to as much as 10^9 per liter in heavily polluted urban areas [10]. Thus, even in relatively clean air, we daily inhale ~5×10^{10} particles, which range in diameter from 1 nm to 1 mm [11]. The probability of the smallest (≤10 nm diameter) and largest particles (>5 μm diameter) depositing in any given breath is ~0.9 (Figure 2). For particles of intermediate size, the probability is less, reaching a minimum of ~0.2 at ~0.5 μm particle diameter (Figure 2). Particles ≥10 μm diameter are deposited predominantly in the extrathoracic airways (the nose and larynx) and the tracheobronchial tree; few reach the alveoli. Bacteria have the same deposition pattern; though most have diameters between 0.2 and 1.0 μm, they are generally attached to dry environmental aerosols or droplets of much larger diameter [12]. Particles ≤5 μm diameter deposit predominantly in the alveoli (Figure 2). However, a significant number of the smallest particles (<0.05 μm diameter) deposit in the tracheobronchial tree (Figure 2).

What is the rate of deposition of large particles on the airway epithelium? Particles ≥1 μm diameter comprise ~0.5% of all atmospheric particles [10]. During mouth breathing, about 90% are deposited per breath, a third of them in the tracheobronchial tree (Figure 2). The total area of

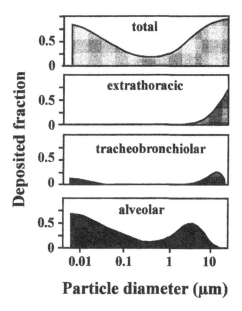

FIGURE 2: Probabilities of particle deposition along the airways during mouth breathing. Deposited fraction is the fraction deposited in a single breath. The term "extrathoracic" is equivalent to "laryngeal." Adapted from refs. [13, 14].

tracheobronchial epithelium is ~4 m^2 [15]. So when mouth breathing, the inhalation of ~5 × 10^{10} particles per day in rural areas corresponds to an average impaction rate of ~1000 large particles per cm^2 of airway surface per day. The corresponding value for heavily polluted air is 200,000 per cm^2 per day.

The impaction rates calculated above are averages for the airway epithelium as a whole. However, for large particles, impaction rates decline dramatically with increasing airway generation. Thus, model calculations [16] indicate that for particles of 11 μm diameter, maximal deposition of 12% occurs in generation 4, declining to 4% in generation 10% and 2% in generation 16. The combined surface area of generation 4 airways is 20 cm^2, of generation 10 is 130 cm^2, and of generation 16 is 1358 cm^2 [17]. So numbers depositing per cm^2 are in the ratio of 100: 5: 0.2 for the three generations. Particles of 1.6 μm diameter deposit predominantly in the smallest airways [13, 16]. Nevertheless, their relative rates of deposition per unit surface also declines with increasing airway generation, being 100:23:4 for generations 4, 10 and 16, respectively [16].

Thus, an exponential increase in combined surface area with increasing airway generation is mainly responsible for particle deposition per unit area being reduced by orders of magnitude with progression from the trachea to the respiratory bronchioles. The secretion of mucus by the epithelium declines accordingly.

Gel-forming mucins are produced by three types of airway epithelial cell. Mucous cells in submucosal glands produce comparatively large amounts under the influence of neurohumoral agents acting on receptors on their basolateral membranes (obviously all glands are submucosal, so the adjective as applied to airway glands expresses the fact that they have short ducts and are therefore immediately beneath the mucosa). Goblet cells in the surface epithelium produce smaller volumes of mucous secretion in response to irritants and autocrine mediators in the ASL. Clara cells in the smallest airways release mucins constitutively [18], but usually not in sufficient quantities to form a detectable gel.

Submucosal glands occur most densely in the nasal cavities and upper airways [19, 20]. During nose breathing in people ~50% of inhaled particles are filtered out in the nose [13], and the percentage is probably considerably higher in many other mammals. In the human tracheobronchial tree, the aggregate volume of glands per cm^2 of airway surface area is greatest in generations 0–4, then declines until they disappear at about generation 8 [21]. Glands are especially numerous at points of bifurcation [21], where increased turbulence results in increased deposition of particles [22]. Goblet cells account for about one in four of the columnar cells of the airway epithelium in the larger airways [23], but decline in frequency with increasing airway generation, and disappear a few generations after the glands [23] (Figure 3). Why the largest airways need both glands and goblet cells is not entirely clear. However, goblet cells represent a low volume rapid-response system whereas glands respond more slowly but can secrete much greater volumes. Also, the two secrete different gel-forming mucins. MUC5B is the predominant glandular mucin and MUC5AC is the main goblet cell mucin [24]. Unfortunately, virtually nothing is known about the comparative functional properties of the two mucins. Mucus secretion by Clara cells combined with phagocytosis by alveolar macrophages and other leukocytes can cope with the particle load in the smallest airways. Should, for any reason, particle deposition increase dramatically in small airways, the resulting inflammation increases the rate of MUC5AC production by Clara cells and they convert to goblet cells [18].

The basic cellular distribution shown in Figure 3 applies to all mammals the size of dogs and larger. However, the smallest mammals studied (mouse and hamster), possess no goblet cells in their tracheobronchial trees [25], and glands are only found at the tracheolaryngeal junction [26]. Rats possess a few small glands [26], but no goblet cells (at least in health) [27]. Most intermediate sized animals (cat, ferret, monkey) possess goblet cells though glands are smaller in individual and aggregate volume than in the larger species [23, 28].

In addition to generating a mucous blanket, there are two other important ways in which airway epithelium alters ASL in response to inhaled insults. First, both glandular and surface epithelia secrete a wide array of anti-microbials, anti-oxidants, anti-proteases and other compounds

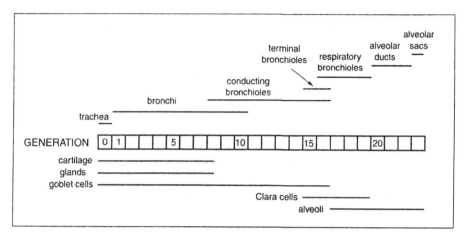

FIGURE 3: Nomenclature of human airways, and distribution of gland-secreting cells and other structures.

that inhibit microbial growth and inactivate toxins. Second, active fluid secretion by the epithelium can increase the volume of ASL and thereby reduce the concentration of dissolved toxins. In large airways of the larger species there is about one gland opening per mm^2 of surface [28, 29], and the maximal secretory rate of individual glands is ~20 nl/min [30]. Glands can therefore add liquid to the airway lumen at a maximal rate of ~2 $\mu l\ min^{-1}\ cm^{-2}$. So, as has been shown experimentally [31], a minute of continuous secretion from all glands approximately triples the depth and volume of ASL. Though mucins in gland secretions may be too dilute to form a gel that can be effectively shifted by cilia, constitutive absorption of liquid by the surface epithelium at a rate of ~0.1 $\mu l\ min^{-1}\ cm^{-2}$ [31–33] concentrates the mucins in the ASL to form a blanket that is moveable (see Figure 4).

The surface epithelium may also secrete liquid in response to neurohumoral and inflammatory stimuli, but at a rate considerably less than the maximal rate achieved by gland secretion [32, 34, 35].

Gland volume secretion and water flows across the surface epithelium are driven by active transepithelial transport of solutes. Active absorption of Na^+ is mainly responsible for liquid absorption; active secretion of Cl^- for liquid secretion. Disease-related changes in these transport processes influence the efficiency of mucociliary clearance by altering the depth of the periciliary sol and the degree of hydration of the mucous blanket.

Toxins that are not neutralized in the ASL may be taken up and destroyed within the epithelial cells themselves. All the columnar cells of airway epithelium are capable of this to some degree,

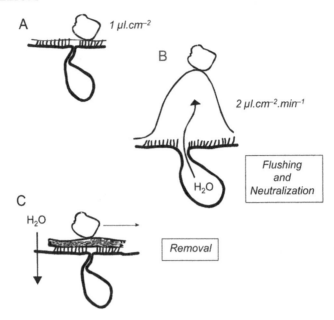

FIGURE 4: Defense functions of large airway epithelia. 1) The ASL consists of two components: a sol around the cilia that lacks gel-forming mucins (the periciliary sol) and a mucous gel lying on the tips of the cilia. In completely healthy airways the gel is thin, incomplete or even absent. 2) In response to irritation (here in the form of a large particle), primary gland secretions dilute any toxins and add a wide range of defensive compounds to the ASL. 3) Constitutive absorption of water across the surface epithelium then concentrates the gland mucins to form (or augment) the mucus gel thereby inducing (or enhancing) mucociliary clearance. In small airways the secretory functions of glands are taken over by the surface epithelium.

but it is the specialty of the Clara cells of the bronchioles. These cells are enriched in cytochrome P450 monooxygenases [36], a family of proteins that metabolize a wide variety of solutes.

In the sections that follow the basic structures and functions of surface and gland epithelia are discussed, with an emphasis on how these epithelia defend the airways, and how these defenses are altered in disease.

·　·　·　·

CHAPTER 2

Surface Epithelium

2.1 OVERALL MORPHOLOGY

In the tracheas and large bronchi of large mammalian species, such as humans, the epithelium is as much as 50 μm in height and is "pseudostratified." Though there are no separate layers of cells (all contact the basement membrane), a stratified appearance is created because different cell types tend to have nuclei at different levels in the epithelium. Columnar cells contact the airway lumen. Quantitatively, much the most important of these are goblet (mucus-secreting) and ciliated cells, with the latter outnumbering the former by ~4:1 in healthy human trachea [23]. Of the non-columnar cells, basal cells are small and either spherical (~8 μm diameter) or squamous. "Intermediate cells" stretch some distance from the basement membrane towards the luminal surface.

With increase in airway generation, the height of the human airway epithelium falls from the maximum of ~50 μm to as little as 5 μm, and it progresses from pseudostratified through simple columnar to cuboidal. The cellular composition also changes. Basal cells account for ~30% of the total in airways >2 mm diameter (generations 0 to 8). After that they decline progressively with increasing generation, accounting for 6% of epithelial cells in airways of diameter <0.5 mm [37]. As shown in Figure 3, Clara cells (non-ciliated non-mucous) replace goblet cells at the transition from conducting to respiratory bronchioles [38]. The loss of goblet cells reflects a drop in the numbers of particles landing on the airway surface. But why are Clara cells, specialized for neutralizing toxic vapors, commoner in small than large airways? The answer may be that velocity of airflow is at least a 100-fold less in the respiratory bronchioles than in the trachea, and at lower velocities lateral diffusion of toxins from the luminal gases into the ASL will increase. Ciliated cells remain constant at ~30–50% of the total in human airways of all sizes [39]. This raises the question of what they are propelling in the mucus-free lower airways. However, contrary to widely held earlier belief [40], the periciliary sol moves towards the mouth at essentially the same rate as the mucous blanket [41].

In other mammalian species, the form and composition of the airway epithelium are dependent almost entirely on airway size, not airway generation [23]. The epithelium of mouse trachea, for instance, has essentially the same cellular composition as that of human bronchioles, not human trachea [42]. The numbers of basal cells decline from about 30% to 40% in the tracheas of species in the size range of rabbits and sheep to 13% in the rat, 8% in the mouse and 6% in the hamster [23]. Similarly, with decrease in tracheal size there is a progressive replacement of goblet cells by Clara cells. Goblet cells are the predominant non-ciliated columnar cell in tracheas of sheep, bonnet and rhesus monkeys, dog, cat, bowhead whale, goat, yak, domestic ox, one-humped camel and pig [23, 31, 43–51]. The same is probably also true of the ferret, assuming the dark cytoplasmic cells described in this species are discharged or immature goblet cells [52]. Guinea pig and rabbit tracheas have a mixture of goblet and Clara cells [53, 54]. In mouse and hamster, goblet cells are completely

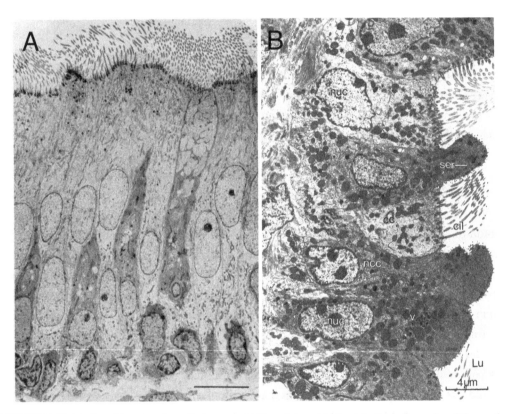

FIGURE 5: Epithelia of large and small airways. A) Pseudostratified epithelium from dog. Most columnar cells are ciliated. The apical portion of a goblet cell with typical mucous granules is present, as are the bases of several other goblet cells. Small basal cells cover most of the basement membrane. Scale bar = 10 μm. Taken from ref. [58]. B) Cuboidal epithelium from mouse. Clara cells comprise 50% of the total. Basal and goblet cells are absent. The histology resembles that of human bronchiole. Nuc = nucleus; cc = ciliated cell; ncc = nonciliated (Clara) cell; cil = cilia; v = secretory vesicle; ser = smooth endoplasmic reticulum; Lu = lumen. Adapted from ref. [42].

replaced by Clara cells [42, 45, 55]. The rat is unusual in that the predominant secretory cell in its trachea is the serous cell [27]. Interestingly, goblet cells are absent or very rare in all horse airways [56], consistent with the paucity of airway glands in this species [57]. It is probable that virtually all large inhaled particles deposit in the complex nasal turbinates of this obligate nose breather.

To summarize, the largest airways are pseudostratified columnar with ciliated, basal and goblet cells being the predominant cell types. By contrast, in airways the size of human respiratory bronchioles, only two major cell types are usually present: ciliated and Clara. These basic histological differences between the epithelia of large and small airways are illustrated in Figure 5.

The nose and upper airways are lined with a mixture of stratified squamous, pseudostratified ciliated, nonciliated columnar and olfactory epithelia [23].

2.2 CELL TYPES

2.2.1 Basal and Intermediate Cells

Basal cells lie on the basement membrane between the columnar cells. They vary from squamous to approximately spherical depending on airway and species [59, 60]. On enzymatic dispersion of dog tracheal epithelium, viable cells became spherical, and the diameter of basal cells averaged 8 μm, whereas ciliated and goblet cells were 10 and 12 μm in average diameter, respectively [58]. Thus, basal cell volume is only ~50% that of ciliated cells and 25% that of mature goblet cells. In situ, the basal cells of sheep trachea, which are approximately spherical, are also only ~8 μm in diameter [60].

Structural evidence convincingly argues that basal cells serve to hold the epithelium in place [60, 61]. They are attached to the neighboring columnar cells by desmosomes, and to the basement membrane by hemidesmosomes from which anchoring filaments penetrate the basement membrane [62]; columnar cells lack hemidesmosomes [62]. Basal cells are also rich in tonofilaments that run between desmosomes and hemidesmosomes. Across tracheas of various species there is an approximately linear relationship between the height of the epithelium and the numbers of basal cells per unit area of basement membrane (Figure 6A). In fact, in the tallest epithelia ~90% of the basement membrane is covered by basal cells (Figure 6B), and the basal poles of the columnar cells are reduced to thin stalks.

Basal cells also function as stem cells, capable of generating the various columnar cell types of the epithelium (see Section 2.4).

Cells that extend towards or reach the lumen, but possess neither cilia nor mucous granules have been referred to variously as intermediate, indifferent, or indeterminate cells. Cytokeratins 5 and 14 are preferentially expressed in basal and intermediate cells, suggesting that the latter are basal cells in the process of developing into columnar cells [37]. For this reason, intermediate cells are sometimes referred to as parabasal cells.

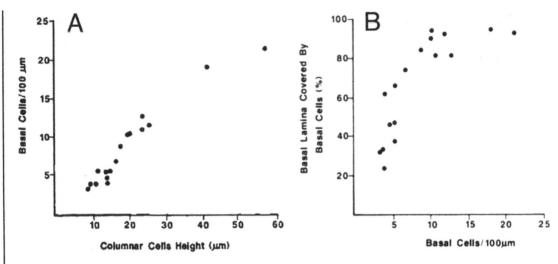

FIGURE 6: Role of basal cells in anchoring the epithelium. A) The numbers of basal cells per unit length of basement membrane increases with epithelial height. B) In the tallest epithelia, basal cells occupy ~90% of the basement membrane area. Points represent 3 tracheas from each of 6 species ranging in size from mouse to sheep. Adapted from ref. [61].

In the epithelium of the epididymis, basal cells stain selectively for COX-1 (cyclooxygenase-1), and about 5% of these send thin projections through tricellular junctions and into the lumen. Here, they sample angiotensin, in response to which they release NO that triggers neighboring cells to secrete protons [63]. COX-1 positive basal cells with luminal projections have been discovered in rat trachea [63]. Their numbers and function are unknown.

2.2.2   Ciliated Cells

In the trachea, bronchi and conducting bronchioles of all species, ciliated cells account for 30% to 80% of the columnar cells [23]. Depending on species, respiratory bronchioles may or may not have ciliated cells [23]. The apical membrane of each ciliated cell contains between 100 and 250 cilia. They are about 7 μm long in the largest airways and 4 μm in the smallest. They are ~200 nm in diameter [64]. There are about 8 cilia per μm^2 of apical membrane corresponding to center-to-center spacing of ~400 nm (i.e., ~200 nm between the surfaces of adjacent cilia) [64]. On the tip of each cilium are ~10 projections about 20 nm long, which are believed to attach to the underside of the mucous gel during mucociliary clearance [27]. The cytoplasm is electron-lucent reflecting a dearth of ribosomes. The apical pole is enriched in mitochondria.

Ciliated cells are probably the key players in transepithelial salt and water transport. Thus, compared to other airway epithelial cell types, their apical membranes are enriched in ion channels necessary for active secretion of Cl⁻ and active absorption of Na⁺. Specifically, these channels are the cystic fibrosis transmembrane conductance regulator (CFTR; a cAMP-activated Cl⁻ channel), ENaC (the epithelial Na⁺ channel) and TMEM16a (probably the major Ca-activated Cl⁻ channel of airway epithelium) [65–68]. Further, between the cilia, the membrane is thrown up into abundant long microvilli, an adaptation that, together with the cilia themselves, will increase the numbers of ion channels per unit area of apical surface. The high numbers of mitochondria are also consistent with active vectorial transepithelial solute transport.

Like primary cilia, airway cilia contain members of the bitter taste receptor family, and bitter compounds increase $[Ca^{2+}]_i$ in airway ciliated cells [69]. The resulting increase in ciliary beat frequency and changes in active transepithelial transport of salts and water defend against the offending compound. Airway cilia also contain acid-sensing ion channels [70].

2.2.3 Goblet Cells

The entire upper two-thirds to four-fifths of mature goblet cells are packed with large (500–2500 nm diameter) [71] electron-lucent granules that contain mucins, predominantly MUC5AC [72]. These granules distend the cells' apices to produce the characteristic goblet shape; immature or discharged goblet cells are more cylindrical. Goblet cells have a comparatively electron-dense cytoplasm associated with large amounts of rough endoplasmic reticulum.

Unlike ciliated cells, goblet cells do not contain detectable levels of CFTR or mRNA for ENaC [66, 67].

It is a little unclear whether immature goblet cells can function as stem cells. Most of the work on airway epithelial turnover and regeneration is done on rodents, where Clara and serous cells are the main secretory cell types.

2.2.4 Clara Cells

As airways decrease in size, goblet cells are replaced by Clara cells, and this latter is the typical non-ciliated columnar cell of the epithelium of respiratory bronchioles in almost all species. Though structurally heterogeneous, Clara cells are characterized by cell apices that protrude into the lumen (Figure 5B), by a small number of small ovoid electron-dense secretory vesicles, by (in most species, but not humans) an abundance of smooth endoplasmic reticulum (SER) in their apices, and by a dearth of microvilli on the apical membrane [73]. In many species Clara cells are enriched with glycogen, which, in the cat, accounts for 40% of the cytoplasmic volume [73].

The SER of Clara cells is enriched in cytochrome P450 monooxygenases [73], a system of enzymes that breaks down a wide variety of inhaled toxins. In addition, Clara cells secrete a number of protective substances such as antileukoproteases [74]. However, perhaps the most abundant secreted protein of Clara cells is CCSP (Clara cell secretory protein) [75]; in CCSP-deficient mice the secretory granules of Clara cells virtually disappear [76]. A variety of anti-oxidant, anti-inflammatory and regenerative roles have been proposed for CCSP [77].

Clara cells contain ENaC mRNA [67], and cultures of Clara cells show active net transepithelial absorption of Na^+ [78]. Chloride secretion is negligible under baseline conditions [78], but can be induced with ATP or β-adrenergic agents [79, 80]. CFTR-like Cl^- channels have been detected electrophysiologically in Clara cell cultures [81], but CFTR is undetectable by immunocytochemistry [66].

In response to injury, Clara cells are able to regenerate ciliated cells and produce goblet cells [18, 82]. Their ability to function as stem cells is inversely related to their maturity as assessed from the numbers of secretory granules [83].

2.2.5 Serous Cells

Serous cells of surface epithelium resemble those of submucosal glands. They are common only in the tracheas of pathogen-free rats, human fetuses, and young hamsters [84], but they are found in small numbers in adult human bronchioles [85]. They are replaced by goblet cells in rats subjected to airway irritation [86]. In human bronchioles, serous cells differ from Clara cells in several ways. First, their apices do not protrude as much. Second, their secretory granules are more numerous (by a factor of four) and more concentrated in the cell apices. Third, the mean diameter of serous cell granules is larger (~0.40 μm for the major axis in serous cells vs. 0.28 μm in Clara cells). Fourth, their apical membranes have more microvilli [85].

The function of serous cells of airway surface epithelium is not known, but by analogy with gland serous cells they may be involved in secretion of liquid and of antimicrobials. They can trans-differentiate into goblet cells in response to injury [87].

2.2.6 Other Cell Types

Neuroendocrine cells (also known as small-granule cells) are usually regarded as part of the APUD (amine, precursor uptake decarboxylase) cell system of endocrine cells that secrete low molecular weight polypeptide hormones [88]. They are generally innervated. Small (100–300 nm diameter) secretory granules in their bases have an opaque periphery surrounding an electron-dense core and contain serotonin, bombesin, and other peptides, as well as monoamines. Neuroendocrine cells are found at all levels of the airways, either individually or in clusters of up to 100; the larger aggregations are known as neuroepithelial bodies. Most, if not all, neuroendocrine cells probably contact the airway lumen. They are commonest at airway bifurcations, contain O_2 receptors, and degranulate in response to hypoxia and hypercapnia. They may, therefore, be involved in local and reflex matching of ventilation and perfusion [89]. It has also been proposed that secretion of gastrin-releasing peptide from neuroendocrine cells plays a role in lung development. Thus, after birth GRP levels in airway epithelium usually drop, but should they stay inappropriately elevated they may cause bronchopulmonary dysplasia [90].

Brush cells are characterized by large apical membrane microvilli containing villin and fimbrin [91]. They are found throughout the airways and alveoli in man and other mammals [91]. They respond to bitter substances by releasing acetylcholine, activating associated sensory nerve terminals, and reflexly inhibiting breathing [92, 93]. In mouse trachea they account for ~1% of epithelial cells [92, 94].

Oncocytes are large mitochondria-rich cells that are very rare in surface epithelium, but somewhat commoner in glands [95, 96]. They may represent the beginnings of cysts or tumors [97]. So-called transitional cells possess both cilia and secretory granules, and presumably represent stages in the development of ciliated cells from either Clara or immature goblet cells. Special-type cells contain small numbers of electron-dense membrane-bound granules in the form of discs or rods (~300 × 50 nm) and have no contact with the lumen. They may be degenerating ciliated cells [98]. The different cell types of airway epithelium, their distinguishing features and probable functions are summarized in Table 1.

Several types of white blood cell are found even in healthy airway epithelium. Lymphocytes are the commonest and their lack of organelles suggests that they are not producing immunoglobulins. They are believed to kill infected epithelial cells, activate other leukocytes, and stimulate survival of epithelial cells via production of growth factors [99]. Globular leukocytes contain very electron-dense homogeneous granules about 600 nm in mean diameter with characteristic cytochemical reactions. They are derived from subepithelial mast cells, migrate into the lumen of inflamed airways, and may be involved in defense against parasitic infections [100]. Dendritic cells are 25–40 μm in length and 2–8 μm wide with two or three slender cytoplasmic processes that probably extend into the airway lumen [101]. They are derived from bone-marrow precursor cells, and present antigen to T lymphocytes [101]. In human airways, there are ~45 neuroendocrine cells for every 10,000 epithelial cells [102].

As reviewed elsewhere [103], the airways contain an intrinsic nervous system. In dog and ferret, it is in several layers (plexuses): in the smooth muscle, around the glands and just below the surface epithelium. In the ventral surface of ferret trachea (i.e. in the absence of smooth muscle) there are ~200 neurons per cm^2 of epithelial surface. The major transmitters in the plexuses are acetylcholine and VIP; in the submucosal plexus of the cat trachea cholinergic varicosities outnumber adrenergic by nine to one. In addition there are sensory nerve terminals within the epithelium itself [104]. In humans these are quite scarce: only about one per mm of basement membrane in cross sections. Nevertheless, substance P released from these terminals is an important regulator of gland secretion both by a direct action and indirectly by activating other nerves in the plexus (see Chapter 3). The activity of the intrinsic plexuses is greatly enhanced by parasympathetic, but not sympathetic input.

CELL TYPE	DISTINCTIVE FEATURES	MAIN FUNCTIONS
	TABLE 1: Airway epithelial cells.	
Basal	Small. Non-columnar. Rich in desmosomes, hemidesmosomes and tonofilaments.	Anchor columnar cells to basement membrane. Stem cells.
Intermediate, indifferent, indeterminate	Non-columnar. Resemble basal cells but project towards lumen.	Basal cells in process of differentiating into columnar cells.
Ciliated	Cilia. Abundant mitochondria.	Mucociliary clearance. Transepithelial salt and water transport.
Goblet	Abundant electron-lucent secretory granules.	Mucus secretion. Stem cells?
Clara cells	Protruding apices. Smooth apical membranes. Abundant SER. Sparse electron-dense secretory granules. High levels of cytochrome P450 monooxygenase (in most species).	Metabolism of toxins. Secretion of protective substances. Transepithelial salt and water transport. Stem cells.
Serous cells	Numerous electron-dense secretory granules.	Secretion of salts and water. Secretion of antimicrobials. Stem cells.
Oncocytes	Abundant mitochondria.	Precancerous?
Brush	Apical membrane brush border.	Chemosensory.
Neuroendocrine cells	Small granules mainly in base of cell. Innervated.	Ventilation/perfusion matching.
Special-type cells	Electron-dense discs or rods.	Degenerating ciliated cells?

2.3   DEVELOPMENT, MAINTENANCE, REGENERATION AND METAPLASIA

In early fetal life, the only type of epithelial cell present in the airways is a non-differentiated columnar cell that shows sparse endoplasmic reticulum, a small Golgi apparatus, no secretory granules and an apical membrane that lacks both microvilli and cilia [105, 106]. In large airways, the first differentiated cell to appear is the neuroendocrine cell, followed by ciliated cells, then secretory cells, with basal cells appearing last [105–107]. All these cell types are thought to arise directly from the undifferentiated columnar cells [107]. In smaller airways, it is unknown whether both ciliated and Clara cells are derived from the undifferentiated primordial cells, or whether ciliated cells derive from Clara as occurs during wound healing [108] and maintenance of adult epithelium [87].

In hamster and monkey, the various differentiated tracheal cell types appear relatively early in fetal life, and their proportions do not change much after birth though they may undergo further differentiation [105, 106, 109]. However, in ferret, mouse and rat there are dramatic changes in the relative numbers of the different cell types after birth [98, 110, 111].

The cell turnover rate of healthy adult airway epithelium is very low, with only ~0.01% to 0.03% of cells entering mitosis per hour, corresponding to labeling indices (LI; the number of cells in the S phase) of 0.1% to 2% [112]. By contrast, LI for stratified squamous epithelia is generally ~10%, and may be as high as 50% in parts of the intestinal epithelium [113]. Estimates of the turnover time for airway epithelium (the hypothetical time needed to double cell numbers in the absence of cell death) range from 20 to 200 days [112]; in oral epithelium it is ~10 days [113].

At such slow turnover rates, it is difficult to identify the cells responsible for routine maintenance of the epithelium. Nevertheless, where basal cells are present they probably play the major role. Thus, Breuer et al. [114] injected [^{3}H]-thymidine into hamsters and prepared autoradiograms of sections from the left intrapulmonary hilar bronchi. About 500,000 cells were examined, and in agreement with earlier workers they found an average LI of ~0.15%. Though basal cells were only 6% of the total, they had the highest LI (~1.5%). Their cell cycle time was 20.6 days and the S-phase of the cell cycle was 7.5 h. The fraction of labeled basal cells decreased with time, while the number of labeled ciliated, secretory and intermediate cells increased. It was concluded that basal cells maintained themselves by self-renewal and also acted as a source of the other cell types.

Recently the role of basal cells in epithelial maintenance has been reinvestigated in transgenic mice by lineage tracing using a Cre-loxP system that allows inducible expression of reporter genes in basal cells and all their progeny [115]. Immediately following induction of the reporter gene, 98% of labeled cells in mouse trachea were identified as basal cells. Over time, however, the label appeared increasingly in both Clara and ciliated cells (Figure 7) [115].

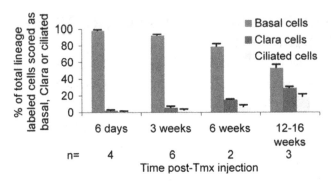

FIGURE 7: Production of ciliated and Clara cells from basal cells. Reporter gene (Lac-Z) expression was induced, and the numbers of positive cells determined at varying times after induction. Ciliated cells were identified by staining for acetylated antitubulin and Clara cells by staining for Clara cell secretory protein. Taken from ref. [115].

The type of progeny generated by basal cells varies with local conditions. Thus, damaging the epithelium with SO_2 led to a much faster transformation of basal into ciliated and Clara cells, and in contrast to basal conditions more ciliated cells were generated than Clara [115].

Also consistent with a role for basal cells as stem cells, multiple studies have shown that purified basal cells can recreate all the cell types of native mucociliary epithelium in a variety of cell culture systems [116].

In respiratory bronchioles, basal cells are absent, and the epithelium consists of only Clara, ciliated and neuroendocrine cells. In response to injury of the epithelium in these airways, there is compelling evidence that Clara cells are the stem cell that not only renews itself but also generates new ciliated cells [108]. Recently, it has been shown using the Cre-loxP lineage tracing system that Clara cells are also responsible for the routine maintenance of mouse bronchiolar epithelium where they not only self-renew but also differentiate into ciliated cells. By contrast, Clara cells in mouse trachea give rise to ciliated cells but show little self-renewal; they are a so-called transiently amplifying population derived from basal cells. However, their capacity for self-renewal increases in response to injury [117]. The Clara cells that function as stem cells seem to be a "variant" sub-population that is resistant to destruction by naphthalene (an agent widely used for the selective destruction of Clara cells) [118].

Serous and Clara cells can both differentiate into goblet cells [18, 119]. Further, there is evidence that during wound healing, immature secretory cells (either serous or Clara) can dedifferentiate and then redifferentiate into all the various cell types of normal airway epithelium [83, 87]. By contrast, mature secretory cells are much less able to alter their phenotype [83]. There is some limited evidence that immature goblet cells of the large airways can also function as stem cells [112].

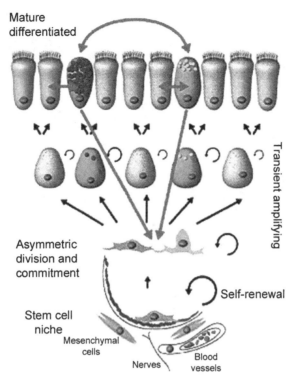

Mature differentiated

Transient amplifying

Asymmetric division and commitment

Self-renewal

Stem cell niche

Mesenchymal cells

Nerves

Blood vessels

FIGURE 8: Cell lineages in pseudostratified airway. Basal cells in various niches within the epithelium are capable of both self-renewal and the generation of parabasal and intermediate cells. These in turn produce the major columnar cell types (upward black arrows). The self-renewing capabilities of these different pools of cells are indicated by the relative size and thickness of the circular arrows. In addition, secretory cells are able to dedifferentiate (downwards red arrows) and join the pool of regenerating cells. Finally, there is transdifferentiation of Clara to goblet and Clara or goblet to ciliated cells (horizontal red arrows). Taken from ref. [87].

Neuroendocrine cells proliferate in response to injury, but can only produce new neuroendocrine cells [118].

For many years, ciliated cells were considered terminally differentiated, and incapable of contributing to the maintenance or regeneration of airway epithelium. Then, in the late 1990s and early 2000s, several studies on mice suggested that they were capable of proliferating and transdifferentiating into Clara cells in response to injury [87]. However, recent lineage mapping studies have shown that ciliated cells do not divide following injury with either naphthalene or SO_2, though they may transiently change their morphology [120].

In summary basal cells may be the main stem cell of pseudostratified airway epithelium under normal conditions. In bronchioles, the Clara cells are responsible for maintaining the epithelium.

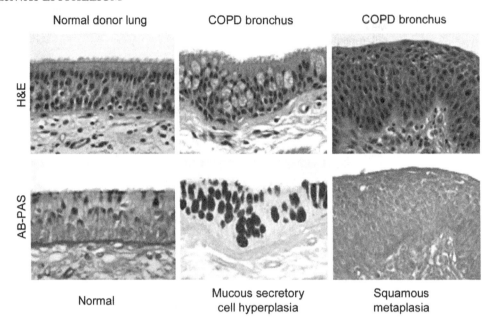

FIGURE 9: Mucous hyperplasia and squamous metaplasia in chronic obstructive pulmonary disease. Top panels stained with hematoxylin and eosin (H&E). Bottom panels stained with Alcian blue—periodic acid Schiff reagent for mucins. Taken from ref. [87].

However, in response to injury, the epithelium shows remarkable plasticity. Not only do basal and Clara cells increase their rates of division, but secretory cells are able to dedifferentiate and then regenerate the other columnar epithelial cell types (Figure 8).

A "niche" is the anatomical and chemical microenvironment in which the stem cell resides [121]. The four currently recognized niches in mouse airways and their associated stem cells are: an unknown cell type in the submucosal gland ducts, basal cells found predominantly in the intercartilaginous zones of the surface epithelium, variant (naphthalene-insensitive) Clara cells associated with neuroendocrine bodies, and variant Clara cells associated with the junctions of bronchioles and alveoli. Stem cells from all these niches can regenerate Clara and ciliated cells of surface epithelium. In addition, cells from the bronchiolar–alveolar niche can regenerate alveolar epithelium [87, 121].

Hyperplasia refers to an increase in numbers of a cell type already present. Metaplasia refers to the appearance of a new cell type. Two main types of remodeling are seen in inflammatory airway disease: mucous hyperplasia/metaplasia and squamous metaplasia (Figure 9).

Goblet cell metaplasia/hyperplasia is characteristic of all inflammatory airway diseases, and can be induced by a variety of insults including tobacco smoke, acrolein, bacterial products, neutrophil elastase, ozone and allergens [122]. However, all these may ultimately act through release of

IL-13 (and activation of STAT6 pathways) and/or activation of the epidermal growth factor receptor (EGFR) [123]. In most cases the major source of IL-13 is probably Th2 lymphocytes, but some cytokines induce IL-13 release from the airway epithelium [123]. As mentioned, goblet cells can be generated from Clara, serous and basal cells. Recent reviews [121, 123] discuss the transcription factors driving mucous metaplasia/hyperplasia. Restoration of the normal epithelia phenotype is by apoptosis and requires downregulation of the anti-apoptotic factor, Bcl-2 [124].

Compared to mucous metaplasia, comparatively little is known about how stratified squamous metaplasia develops [125]. In vivo and in vitro it can be induced by depletion of retinoic acid and reversed by retinoic acid supplementation [126]. A number of inflammatory cytokines have also been implicated in its genesis [127].

2.4   BARRIER FUNCTION

The two major functions of epithelia are to provide a barrier and to bring about net transepithelial transport of solutes (and water). Depending on the form of the barrier, transepithelial solute transport can produce very different results [128]. "Tight" epithelia (e.g., frog skin) have low salt and water permeability, and active transepithelial salt transport generates and maintains solutions of widely different NaCl concentrations on either side of the epithelium. "Leaky" epithelia, by contrast, have high osmotic and ionic permeabilities and are incapable of maintaining significant concentration differences between the serosal and mucosal bathing media. Instead, vectorial solute transport sets up osmotic differences between the unstirred layers on either side of the tissue that drive absorption or secretion of fluid that is virtually isosmotic with the bathing media [129]. Airway epithelium is moderately leaky to ions. Its high osmotic permeability [130–132] predicts isosmotic fluid absorption (or secretion) [133, 134]. Net flows of salt and water across airway epithelium have never been determined simultaneously. However, in epithelial sheets from the same dog tracheas, aminophylline induced net volume secretion of 137 ± 29 nl cm^{-2} min^{-1} and net Cl$^-$ secretion of 1.44 ± 0.50 μEq cm^{-2} h^{-1} [135]. The ratio of these two values yields a Cl$^-$ concentration in the secreted liquid of 175 ± 71 mEq/l, of which the best that can be said is that it is not inconsistent with isosmolarity!

The transepithelial electrical resistance (R_{te}) is an index of leakiness to ions. It is readily determined from the deflection in transepithelial voltage (V_{te}) in response to current pulses across the epithelium. For airway epithelia, R_{te} ranges from 200 to 1000 Ω cm^2 [136], somewhere in the middle of the range for epithelia in general (5–50,000 Ω cm^2). This wide variation in R_{te} across epithelia is due mainly to differences in the intrinsic leakiness of the tight junctions or in the length of tight junctions per unit area of epithelium (i.e., the size of the cells) [128]; transcellular resistance (the sum of the resistances of the apical and basolateral cell membranes) varies comparatively little.

In general, leakiness of tight junctions to small uncharged hydrophilic solutes parallels their leakiness to ions. More specifically, in dog tracheal epithelium the passive transepithelial fluxes of Na^+ and Cl^- (i.e., the fluxes in the direction opposite to their active transport) both bear linear relationships to the fluxes of mannitol [137], a compound believed to move solely through the paracellular pathway.

Most studies of non-electrolyte permeation across epithelia conclude that there are many small and a few very large pores. In T_{84} and Caco-2 cells (cell lines with R_{te} similar to airway epithelium) the fluxes of wide range of polyethylene glycols (PEG) revealed a predominant paracellular pathway with a restrictive pore radius of ~4.5 Å and a minor pathway with a pore radius >> 7.4 Å [138]. In dog tracheal epithelium, a comparison of the transepithelial fluxes of a variety of radioactive solutes ranging in size from water to inulin also suggested two populations of pores. In this case, the estimated radii were 6 and 250 Å, and the small pores outnumbered the large by ~100,000:1 [139]. Morphological damage to the epithelium led to an increase in radius of the large pores without change in the small [139]. It is tempting to speculate that the small pores lie in healthy tight junctions, and the large are caused by dead or dying cells. So-called tricellular junctions, where one tight junction fuses with another, have also been proposed as the site of the large pores [140]. The permeation cut-off for the small pores occurs at about the size of sucrose. Thus, ions, sugars and amino acids will pass but oligosaccharides and oligopeptides will not. However, the presence of a small population of large pores means that there is a finite paracellular permeability to solutes as large as proteins, though the mathematical model of Man et al. suggests that the permeability to albumen (44 kDa) is only about one-fiftieth that to mannitol [139].

Tight junctional structure has been analyzed by freeze fracture in airway epithelium of several species. In general there are from 4 to 26 parallel strands per tight junction with an average of 7–11 (depending on species). The combined depth of the strands is 0.35–0.5 μm [141–143]. There are subtle differences in the structure of the tight junctions between different cell types [141]. Across epithelia, there is a rough correlation between the numbers of strands and the leakiness of tight junctions to ions [144]. In secretory epithelia such as airway submucosal glands [145], or highly absorptive epithelia such as that of the proximal tubule [146], there are considerably fewer strands. This promotes high rates of transepithelial fluid flow by enhancing passive flows of ions down their electrochemical gradients. The strand numbers for airway surface epithelium are consistent with moderate tightness and fairly low rates of fluid transfer. Thus, fluid absorption across proximal tubular epithelium ranges from 40 to 230 μl cm^{-2} h^{-1} [147], whereas airway epithelium absorbs at ~5 μl cm^{-2} h^{-1} [32].

There is a considerable literature on the breakdown of tight junctional integrity in response to inhalation of atmospheric pollutants such as SO_2, NO_2, ozone and cigarette smoke. Aside from such overt toxicity, there are four basic ways in which paracellular permeability of airway epithelium may be increased. First, tight junctions may open transiently, and alter their ion selectivity, in response to a number of inflammatory mediators. Second, inflammatory mediators may cause slow and progressive loss of tight junctional organization. Third, during inflammatory extravasation, elevation of subepithelial hydrostatic pressure may dilate the lateral intercellular spaces and tear open tight junctions. Fourth, transepithelial migration of leukocytes in large numbers is associated with marked dilation of tricellular junctions.

In the first indication that inflammatory mediators could alter the permeability of airway tight junctions, isolated segments of guinea pig tracheas were instilled with horseradish peroxidase, which appeared in the lateral intercellular spaces of animals given aerosols of histamine or methacholine but not those given control saline [148]. In other studies, when tachykinins were added to dog tracheal epithelium, active Cl^- secretion increased but V_{te} paradoxically dropped for ~20 sec before increasing. Replacement of Cl^- by large organic anions reduced the size of the transient decrease in V_{te}. It was concluded that the decrease in V_{te} was caused by increased permeability of the tight junctions to Cl^- [149]. In rabbit trachea, ATP may also decrease the Cl^- conductance of the tight junctions [150]. The β-adrenergic agent, albuterol, increases mannitol flux across primary cultures of human tracheal epithelium [151].

Recently, the effect of histamine on paracellular permeability has been reinvestigated [152]. Primary cultures of human tracheal epithelium from patients with cystic fibrosis were treated with amiloride. Under these circumstances, there is essentially no active transepithelial ion transport and V_{te} is virtually zero, allowing the relative permeability of the paracellular pathway to Na^+ and Cl^- (P_{Na}/P_{Cl}) to be determined from dilution potentials. Addition of histamine halved R_{te} and increased P_{Na}/P_{Cl}. Both unidirectional transepithelial fluxes of Na^+ increased, but Cl^- fluxes were not affected. Further, the numbers of lateral intercellular spaces into which La^{3+} penetrated was increased by histamine. The actions of histamine were Ca-dependent and transient, lasting about 6 min.

One of the physiological consequences of changes in paracellular permeability and ion selectivity is that they will influence transepithelial water transport. As described in detail later, active absorption of Na^+ is the main vectorial transport process operating across airway surface epithelia. Cl^- follows passively driven by the resulting V_{te}, and water follows the NaCl by osmosis. By increasing the Na^+ permeability of the paracellular pathway, histamine will reduce NaCl (and water) absorption by shunting Na^+ back toward the lumen. The resulting increase in the volume of airway surface liquid could facilitate mucociliary clearance.

In contrast to these transient effects of inflammatory mediators, a combination of interferon-γ (INF-γ) and tumor necrosis factor-α (TNF-α) caused R_{te} of primary cultures of human tracheal epithelium to drop to nearly zero with a half-time of ~24 h. This drop was associated with an equivalent increase in permeability to 2000-kDa dextran, a profound loss of tight junctional strands, and loss of ZO-1 from the region of the tight junctions. Recovery was slow with a half-time of ~8 h [143]. The use of selective pharmacological agents suggested that these effects were mediated by protein kinase C [143]. Interleukin-ß also has slow effects on tight junctional permeability, but of lesser magnitude than those induced with the combination of INF-γ and TNF-α [143].

Applying a positive hydrostatic pressure to the luminal surface of epithelia does not much alter their hydraulic conductivity [153]. However, applying a positive pressure to the serosal side dilates the LIS, opens up tight junctions, and dramatically increases the permeability to water and all solutes. Bulk flows of water and solute toward the lumen ensue [153]. With airway epithelia in vitro, such effects are seen with pressures as low as 5 cm H_2O [154, 155]. In rats, stimulation of the vagal nerves creates "neurogenic inflammation" of the airways [156]. If the blood contains dextran blue, the tracheal wall turns blue from extravasation, and dextran blue and other high molecular weight blood-borne markers appear in the tracheal lumen [157]. However, if a hydrostatic pressure of 5 cm H_2O is applied to the lumen of a perfused segment of trachea, on stimulating the vagi the tracheal wall still turns blue but dextran blue no longer appears in the lumen [157]. Hydrostatic pressures in capillaries and venules are generally considerably higher than 5 cm H_2O (3.5 mm Hg). We suggest therefore that inflammatory extravasation causes interstitial hydrostatic pressures immediately beneath the airway epithelium to increase sufficiently to disrupt tight junctions and drive plasma into the lumen.

Small numbers of neutrophils may migrate across the epithelium without causing significant increase in permeability; the tight junctions open to let the individual neutrophils through and then promptly reseal [158]. However, with increased traffic there may be a continuous flow of neutrophils, the tight junctions do not have time to reseal, the epithelial cells are pushed apart and large wounds result [158]. Tricellular junctions are the preferred sites for neutrophil migration [159]. Being more porous than regular junctions, they are not only easier for neutrophils to disrupt but chemotactic agents released into the lumen will also diffuse preferentially across them.

The paracellular permeability also depends on the cellular composition of the epithelium. Mucous metaplasia is associated with a drop in R_{te} [160], probably related to differences in tight junctional structure in goblet vs. ciliated cells [141]. It would be surprising if squamous metaplasia did not also confer altered barrier function.

In an interesting study, Vermeer et al. [161] describe a mechanism whereby airway epithelium senses breakdown of its own barrier function, and initiates the necessary repair processes. Thus, in primary cultures of the human tracheal epithelium, epidermal growth factor receptors (EGFR) are restricted to the basolateral membrane. In addition, the cells secrete heregulin-α, a ligand of the EGFR, into the ASL. When tight junctions are intact and the epithelium undamaged, ligand and receptor are separated. However, when tight junctions are opened or cells are lost, heregulin-α can reach its receptor and promote wound healing. To test this hypothesis, an area of cells was scraped off, and the rate of wound healing measured. This was slowed when either a neutralizing antibody to heregulin-α or an EGFR antagonist were present, but accelerated by recombinant heregulin-α.

2.5   MUCUS SECRETION

Mucins are large proteins (up to several MDa) defined by tandem repeats of amino acid sequences rich in serine and threonine, to which are attached large branched carbohydrate structures that constitute approximately 70% to 80% of the molecular weight [6, 24, 72]. On average there are about 30 oligosaccharides side-chains per 100 amino acids. The highly variable structure and content of these side-chains helps mucins perform one of their major functions: the binding of pathogens [162].

At least twenty-two mucin (*MUC*) genes are known, of which ~16 are expressed in the airways [163]. Functionally, airway mucins can be divided into three classes. First, there are those that are secreted, polymerize, and form gels. Second, a large number of mucins are tethered to membranes via a single hydrophobic transmembrane sequence. The extracellular glycosylated moieties of these membrane-tethered mucins form the predominant component of the glycocalyx in all cells. On binding pathogens, membrane-tethered mucins activate intracellular signaling pathways that trigger a range of immune responses. Their extracellular domains can be released by cleavage near the transmembrane domain either by proteases or by autocatalysis [6]. These moieties may contribute up to 10% of the mucus blanket [6], but it is unknown how they affect its viscoelastic and antimicrobial properties. The third type of mucin, MUC7, is small (125 kDa) [164] and restricted to gland serous cells [165]. It is secreted but does not polymerize or form gels [166]. Abundant in saliva, this mucin may serve primarily an antimicrobial function [167].

The gel-forming mucins of the airways are MUC2, 5AC, 5B, 6, 8 and 19. MUC5AC is the major mucin of airway goblet cells [168, 169], but is also found at low levels in submucosal glands [170]. MUC5B is the predominant gel-forming mucin of gland mucous cells, but is also found at low levels in goblet and Clara cells of surface epithelium [18, 168, 169]. Together, MUC5AC and MUC5B account for at least 90% of mucins in the airway mucous gel [24]. MUC19 is found predominantly in glands [171], MUC2 in a subpopulation of goblet cells [168], MUC6 at low levels in surface epithelium [172], and MUC8 at low levels in both glands and surface epithelium [168, 173]. MUC2 mRNA is upregulated in airway epithelial cultures by various inflammatory mediators [174]. However, this mucin could not be detected in sputum from either healthy or diseased airways [24].

Individual molecules of MUC5AC average 2–3 MDa in molecular weight, and are linked end-to-end within the cell by S—S bonds to form polymers of up to 50 MDa in weight and 10 μm in length [24]. Most of the carbohydrate side-chains end in sialic acid residues, and many of the sugar moieties are sulfated [162]. Binding of these negative charges to Ca^{2+} allows the mucin to be stored in highly condensed form within secretory granules [175]. On release, the same fixed negative charges mediate a Donnan equilibrium process that expands the granule contents by ~1000-fold within 10 sec [176]. Other gel-forming mucins undoubtedly resemble MUC5AC in their structure, intracellular processing, packaging, and release.

The following membrane-tethered mucins are expressed in the airways: MUC1, 4, 11, 13, 15, 16, 18, 20, 21, and 22 [163]. However, only MUC1, 4, 16 and 18 are known to have significant functions. MUC1 and MUC4 are found predominantly on the apical membrane of ciliated cells [168, 177]. The former extends ~100 nm from the cell surface and is found on microvilli; the later extends ~300 nm and is found on cilia [177]. Cilia are 200 nm wide and 200 nm apart. Thus, the region between the cilia and microvilli is filled with the densely packed extracellular moieties of MUC1 and MUC4 that create an effective mesh size that excludes particles larger than ~25 nm [177]. It has been proposed that the negative charges on the mucins repel one another to create nearly frictionless interactions among the beating cilia. It was originally suggested that MUC16 was synthesized by ciliated cells and played a similar role in the periciliary liquid as MUC1 and MUC4 [177]. However, subsequent immunocytochemical studies show it to be present on cilia but absent from the cytoplasm of ciliated cells. Instead it is found in goblet cells and mucous gland cells and in the mucous blanket [168, 178]. It seems probable therefore that it is secreted by goblet and mucous cells and then adheres to the cilia.

Binding of pathogens by membrane-tethered mucins activates signaling pathways involved in airway defense [6]. For instance, binding of Pseudomonas by MUC1 inhibits TLR signaling, and during inflammation this mucin is upregulated by TNF-α. It may therefore play a key role in the resolution of pulmonary inflammation [163]. Domains in MUC4 that resemble the receptor-binding portions of epidermal growth factor interact with EGFR to potentiate the wound healing response of airway epithelium [179]. MUC18 binds *Mycoplasma pneumonia* and non-typeable *Haemophilus influenza*, and its expression is increased in asthma and by treatment with IL-13 [180].

Goblet cell secretion has been measured in several ways. The rate of discharge of individual granules from living goblet cells has been studied microscopically [181]. Following stimulation with secretagogues, tissues can be fixed and the levels of mucin remaining in goblet cells determined by Alcian blue/PAS staining of conventional histological sections [182]. Another commonly used approach is to measure release of radioactively-labeled high molecular weight glycoconjugates from airways that lack glands or from primary cultures of airway surface epithelium [183]. Kim has developed primary cultures of hamster tracheal epithelium that consist of >90% goblet cells [184]. The radiolabeled material so measured is often assumed to represent gel-forming mucins released from goblet cell mucous granules. However, it could also contain constitutive secretions (i.e., non-granular) or released glycocalyx. Neutrophil elastase, for instance, doubles the rate of release of radiolabeled high molecular weight glycoconjugates from cultures of hamster tracheal epithelium without any apparent degranulation, but with a loss of ~50% of the mucin associated with the glycocalyx [185].

Cholinergic and adrenergic nerve fibers have been found in close proximity to goblet cells of surface epithelium [186], and surface epithelium contains adrenergic and cholinergic receptors

[187, 188]. Despite this, goblet cell discharge in humans, cats, cows, and hamsters is usually refractory to both adrenergic and cholinergic agonists [18, 189]. By contrast, in rats and guinea pigs, vagal stimulation causes loss of PAS-positive material from goblet cells [182, 190], an effect apparently mediated by substance P and acetylcholine in combination [182].

ATP is perhaps the most potent direct secretagogue of goblet cells [18, 189], and it has been shown recently that this agent is released from epithelial cells into the airway lumen by mechanical strain [191]. Other agents that induce goblet cell degranulation in vivo include leukotrienes, prostaglandin $F_{2\alpha}$, substance P, histamine, lipopolysaccharide, bacterial proteases, PAF, stretch, and extremes of pH [192, 193]. Though human neutrophil elastase releases predominantly glycocalyx from primary cultures of hamster tracheal epithelium [185], it degranulates guinea pig airway goblet cells in vivo [194], and releases MUC5AC from well-differentiated primary cultures of human bronchial epithelial cells via a protein kinase C-mediated mechanism [195].

Degranulation of goblet cells in response to ATP has been studied by video microscopy of human and dog airway epithelium in explant culture [71, 181]. Baseline rates of degranulation were ~0.05 granules discharged per min. In the usual response to ATP, after a delay of ~5 sec, the frequency of degranulation events increased to a maximum of ~100 per min within ~10 sec, and then declined within seconds to a rate of ~5 per min (see Figure 10). About half the granules were discharged during this initial rapid transient response.

Macrolide antibiotics inhibit the goblet cell discharge and neutrophil migration induced by lipopolysaccharide (LPS) in vivo [196]; it is unclear whether LPS directly stimulates goblet cell discharge or whether this is caused by the neutrophil migration. Dexamethasone likewise has been shown to inhibit the release of goblet cell mucins in response to antigen challenge [197].

Many studies [18], indicate that ATP, and probably most other mediators, stimulate goblet cell discharge by the classic phospholipase-C pathway. Thus, the ATP receptor is coupled to phospholipase-C (PLC) via GTP-binding proteins sensitive to pertussis toxin. Activation of PLC then generates IP_3 and diacylglycerol (DAG). The IP_3 releases Ca^{2+} and the DAG activates protein kinase C, with nPKCε being the major isoform of involved. Consistent with the lack of effect of adrenergic agents and adrenergic nerve stimulation [198], elevation of intracellular cAMP with permeable analogues of cAMP, forskolin, or phosphodiesterase inhibitors is without effect on goblet cell granule discharge [198, 199].

Clara cells show little or no staining for mucins, but constitutively secrete MUC5B. With inflammatory stimulation, production of MUC5B is upregulated 2- to 5-fold, while MUC5AC production increases up to 100-fold. Mucin production now exceeds secretion, secretory granules appear and the Clara cells become transformed into goblet cells [18].

In well-differentiated primary cultures of human tracheal epithelium, mucins are also secreted in the form of exosomes [200]. Derived from endosomes, these membrane-bound bodies

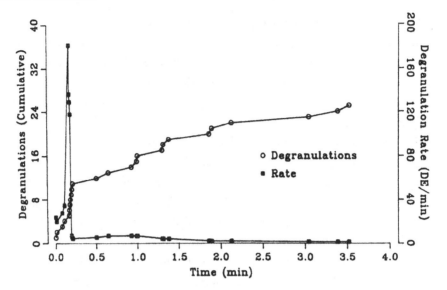

FIGURE 10: Goblet cell discharge in response to mucosal ATP. Representative cell in an explant of dog tracheal epithelium. Plots show cumulative number of granules released, or the rate of "degranulation events," DE/min, as determined on living tissue by video-microscopy. Taken from ref. [181].

have diameters of 30–100 nm, and are enriched in MUC1, MUC4 and MUC16. Sialic acid on the carbohydrate side chains of these mucins confers on exosomes a potent neutralizing action against human influenza virus. It seems probable that exosomes are secreted by ciliated rather than goblet cells.

2.6   MEDIATOR RELEASE AND BREAKDOWN

Bacteria or viruses that deposit on the airway surface bind to toll-like receptors (TLR), membrane-tethered mucins, or other receptors on the apical membrane. In addition, following internalization, viral RNA binds to endosomal TLRs. Signaling pathways are thereby activated that induce the secretion of mucins, antimicrobials and other agents across the apical membrane and of a wide variety of chemokines and cytokines across the basolateral [201]. Many inflammatory products and neurohumoral mediators (e.g., neutrophil elastase) also induce secretion [202]. Even under baseline conditions, the epithelium shows considerable secretory activity. In one recent study, the ASL over primary cultures of human tracheal epithelium was subjected to two-dimensional gel electrophoresis. One hundred and seventy-five spots were detected that represented isomers of 54 proteins [203]. In a second such study, 134 proteins were detected [204]. In a third, fifty-five mucin-associated proteins were found in a high molecular weight fraction of ASL [205].

Mediators have been demonstrated in native epithelium by immunocytochemistry, or their mRNA detected by PCR or FISH. The components of lavage have been measured, but these could come from surface epithelium, glands or even the submucosa. Many compounds have been demonstrated in cultured airway epithelial cells or the medium bathing them. However, some caution should be exercised in extrapolating these findings to native epithelium; the gene expression of even well-differentiated cultures is altered. For instance, primary cultures of human tracheal epithelium release lactoferrin and lysozyme [206], but in native airways these compounds can only be demonstrated in serous gland cells [207, 208]. More recently, gene expression profiling showed that of about 30,000 genes measured, ~20% showed a greater than two-fold differences in expression between well-differentiated primary cultures and native epithelium. Further, some genes were expressed in cultured cells but not native epithelium, and vice versa [209]. These problems are exacerbated when primary cultures are grown under suboptimal conditions, or when airway epithelial cell lines are used; most of the latter do not even form tight junctions [210].

Table 2 provides a list of biologically active compounds (other than mucins) secreted across the apical membrane of airway surface epithelium, either native or cultured. Most of these compounds are also secreted by glands, often in greater amounts than the surface epithelium, and generally by serous rather than mucous cells.

At least ten of the compounds listed in Table 2 are antimicrobial. Some are secreted constitutively (e.g., hBD-1); most are inducible (e.g., hBD-2) [212]. They kill by several different mechanisms, so they often show synergy [235]. In addition, the glands secrete some antimicrobials, such as lactoferrin and lysozyme, not produced to any significant degree by the surface epithelium. Clearly, the antimicrobials of ASL constitute a highly dynamic system well able to cope with a wide range of bacterial insults [236, 237].

A large number of the bactericidal peptides secreted by airway epithelium are small with C-terminal domains that are cationic at physiological pH and bind to negative charges in the bacterial wall. Hydrophobic domains then insert in the bacterial membrane, and aggregate to form pores that permeabilize and kill the bacteria [238]. Beta-defensins, cathelicidins (of which LL-37 is the only form in humans), elafin, hepcidin, the chemokine, CCL20, and the interferon-inducible cytokines, CXCL9 (MIP), CXCL10 (IP-10) and CXCL11 (I-TAC) belong to this general class of antimicrobials [202, 239].

Most of the cationic antimicrobials have additional effects on innate and induced immunity. Thus, hBD-1, hBD-2 and CCL20 all stimulate the migration of T-cells and immature dendritic cells by activating their CC6 receptors [240–242]. In addition to its bactericidal action, LL-37 contributes to host defense by binding to and neutralizing bacterial LPS (endotoxin), by enhancing proliferation and wound healing of airway epithelial cells, by stimulating epithelial cytokine release,

TABLE 2: Compounds released into ASL by airway epithelium.

COMPOUND	CELL TYPE	IN GLANDS?	FUNCTION	REF
Human beta-defensin-1 and hBD-2	?	Y	Antimicrobial	[211, 212]
Cathelicidin (LL-37)	?	Y	Antimicrobial	[213]
Hepcidin	Culture	?	Antimicrobial	[214]
Lipocalin-1 (Von Ebner's gland protein, siderocalin)	Ciliated	?	Antimicrobial?	[215]
Heregulin	Culture	?	EGFR ligand	[161]
CCL20	?	?	Antimicrobial	[216]
Interferon-inducible cytokines CXCl9, CXCL10 and CXCL11	?	?	Antimicrobial	[217–219]
S100 proteins	?	Y	Antimicrobial	[220]
SPLUNC1	Ciliated	Y	Surfactant activity inhibits Pseudomonas biofilm formation	[221]
LPLUNC	Goblet	Y	Antimicrobial	[222]
Lactoperoxidase (LPO)	Goblet	Y	Antimicrobial in combination with SCN and H_2O_2	[223]

	CELL			
COMPOUND	TYPE	IN GLANDS?	FUNCTION	REF
Hyaluronan	Culture	?	Immobilizes lactoperoxidase Stimulates ciliary motion	[224]
H_2O_2	Ciliated	?	Helps generate HOSCN, a potent antimicrobial agent	[225]
ATP	Ciliated Goblet Clara?	?	Inhibits Na absorption Stimulates Cl secretion & mucin release Increases ciliary beat frequency	[226]
Secretory component; IgA, IgM	Serous Ciliated	Y	Antibody	[227]
Clara cell secretory protein (CC16, CC10, uteroglobulin)	Clara	N?	Antioxidant Immunosuppression Anti-inflammatory	[77]
SLPI	Goblet Clara	Y	Secretory leukocyte protease inhibitor	[74]
Elafin	Goblet	Y	Secretory leukocyte protease inhibitor Antimicrobial	[228]

TABLE 2: (*continued*)

	TABLE 2: *(continued)*			
COMPOUND	**CELL TYPE**	**IN GLANDS?**	**FUNCTION**	**REF**
Cystatin C	Goblet	Y	Cysteine protease inhibitor	[228]
Interferon-β	Culture	?	Anti-viral	[229]
NO	?	?	Manifold	[230]
Trefoil Factor family peptides	Goblet	Y	Mucus rheology Epithelial remodeling	[231]
Surfactant proteins A, B and D	Ciliated	Y	Surfactant activity Antimicrobial	[232]
Prostasin	Culture	?	Regulates active Na^+ absorption	[233]
Serpin protease nexin-1 (PN-1)	Culture	?	Inhibits prostatin	[234]

and by promoting apoptosis of infected cells [243, 244]. Elafin's primary function is inhibition of neutrophil elastase [245].

Lipocalin-2 (siderocalin) kills bacteria by binding their siderophores and thereby starving them of iron [246]. In mouse airways, infection with Klebsiella results in its appearance in Clara and ciliated cells, and knock-out of siderocalin greatly increases sensitivity to bacterial infection [247].

S100 proteins, originally described from skin, have been demonstrated in nasal surface epithelium and glands and in nasal lavage [220]. They are down-regulated in chronic rhinosinusitis suggesting that they may play a causative role in this disease [220]. The mechanism behind their antimicrobial activity is unknown.

Lactoperoxidase (LPO) and H_2O_2 are involved in the production of HOSCN, another potent antimicrobial in ASL. H_2O_2 is produced by the dual oxidases DUOX1 and DUOX2, isoforms of the NADPH oxidase, strongly expressed at the apical pole of ciliated cells in the airways [248]. Lactoperoxidase is secreted mainly by glands but also by goblet cells of the surface epithelium [223].

It catalyzes the reaction of SCN$^-$, secreted by the surface epithelium (see Section 2.8.15), with H$_2$O$_2$ to produce HOSCN. This then kills by oxidizing sulfhydryl groups [249].

Hyaluronan in ASL is probably derived mainly from connective tissues. However, it is secreted by cultured airway epithelial cells [250]. Binding of hyaluronan to receptors on cilia increases ciliary beat frequency [224]. In addition, hyaluronan binds LPO, thereby preventing its removal by mucociliary clearance [251]. Hyaluronan also binds kallikrein [251], produced by glands [252]. In its bound form, kallikrein is inactive. But, in response to reactive oxygen species, hyaluronan breaks down, and kallikrein is released to produce kinins that cause bronchoconstriction [251].

The PLUNC (palate, lung and nasal epithelium clone) family has nine members, two of which are expressed in the airways. SPLUNC1 (short PLUNC1) is found in Clara cells of surface epithelium and, at significantly higher levels, in mucous cells of glands. LPLUNC1 (long PLUNC1), by contrast, is found in goblet cells of surface epithelium and at somewhat higher levels in serous cells of glands [253]. The function of LPLUNC1 in airways is obscure, but SPLUNC1 has surface-active properties that inhibit Pseudomonas biofilm formation [254]. SPLUNC1 also binds to ENaC and prevents its cleavage and activation by serine proteases. It may therefore act as a "volume sensor" that by changes in its concentration can regulate ENaC activity and the volume of ASL [255].

Clara cell secretory protein (CCSP), also known as CC16, CC10 or uteroglobulin, is abundant in Clara cells and is a potent immunosupressor and anti-inflammatory agent [256].

Surfactant proteins A, B and D (but not C) are expressed in ciliated cells of nasal mucosa and in serous cells of nasal glands [232, 257]. Surfactant protein D has also been found in goblet and Clara cells of tracheobronchial epithelium [257]. SPA and D, members of the collectin family, aggregate microorganisms and target them for phagocytosis [258].

SLPI and elafin are potent inhibitors of neutrophil serine proteases [245]. They also show anti-microbial and anti-inflammatory properties, and inhibit the stimulation of mucin secretion by neutrophil elastase [259]. In mice, there is thirty times as much SLPI mRNA in glands as in surface epithelium [260]. Recently, the cysteine protease inhibitor, cystatin C, has been localized to goblet cells and glands of the human nasal sinus [228].

Trefoil factor family peptides are secreted mainly from mucous cells of glands but also from goblet cells of surface epithelium. In addition to binding to mucins and increasing the viscosity of mucus [261], they are involved in the transdifferentiation of Clara and serous cells into goblet cells, as well as in the production of ciliated from non-differentiated squamous cells [231].

Polymeric IgA (pIg) from plasma cells binds to receptors (pIgR) on epithelial basolateral membranes. Together with a portion of this receptor (the secretory component) the pIgA is then transcytosed and secreted into the lumen [262]. Though this system has been most studied in the gut, it is also present in airway surface epithelium [263], and alterations in the amount of IgA

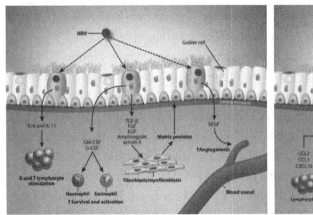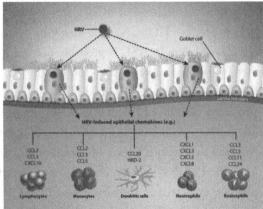

FIGURE 11: Cytokines released across the basolateral membrane of airway epithelium following viral infection. Taken from ref. [269].

transported are believed to contribute to the pathology of both chronic obstructive pulmonary disease (COPD) and asthma [227, 264].

ATP is a potent autocrine regulator of airway epithelial function. It is secreted into the ASL by several routes, of which the most important may be a connexin/pannexin-like channel in the apical membrane of ciliated cells [226]. Within the ASL it is broken down by membrane-bound endonucleases. Under baseline conditions, the resulting steady state ATP concentration in ASL of ~5–20 nM is below the physiological threshold [265]. However, in response to shear stress and other mechanical stimuli, ATP levels in ASL increase transiently to 100–1000 nM. This activates P2Y2 receptors and the resulting increase in $[Ca^{2+}]_i$ stimulates goblet cell discharge, ciliary beat frequency and active Cl^- secretion, while inhibiting active Na^+ absorption [191, 265, 266]. A dramatic enhancement of mucociliary clearance results [267]. Though the initial release of ATP is probably from ciliated cells, more is added during discharge of mucin from goblet cells [268], where ATP is involved in mucin packaging. Adenosine, a major breakdown product of ATP, also enhances mucociliary clearance by activating apical membrane G-protein coupled receptors, elevating intracellular cAMP and stimulating CFTR-dependent Cl^- secretion [266].

In addition to adding substances to the ASL, airway epithelium responds to a wide variety of stimuli by generating chemokines and cytokines that are released across the basolateral membrane [269]. As illustrated in Figure 11, at least twenty cytokines are released following infection by human rhinovirus alone. They stimulate B and T lymphocytes, activate neutrophils and eosinophils, induce fibroblasts to lay down matrix protein, stimulate angiogenesis, and attract a wide variety of leukocytes to the epithelium.

Arachidonic acid metabolites, generated by cyclooxygenase, lipoxygenase and cytochrome P450 monooxygenases are another important class of mediators released by airway epithelium [270]. Between species, there are major differences in the relative importance of the various arachidonic acid metabolic pathways. Further, for the same species, the relative expression of these pathways varies substantially between native epithelium, isolated cells and cell cultures. Native human epithelium differs from that of many species in having comparatively low cyclooxygenase activity and high 15-lipoxygenase activity. Bradykinin and platelet-activating factor are two of the more important mediators inducing production of arachidonic acid metabolites. PGE_2 and PGD_2 are quantitatively the most important of the cyclooxygenase products. The former has a variety of pro-inflammatory and defense actions. It is also a potent stimulator of active Cl^- secretion, at least in dog tracheal epithelium [271]. The bronchoconstrictor, $PGF2\alpha$, is also released in appreciable quantities, predominantly across the basolateral membrane. The major lipoxygenase products are LTB_4 and LTC_4, both of which stimulate epithelial ion transport and mucus secretion [272]. In addition, LTB_4 is a potent chemoattractant agent [273], and LTC_4 a potent vasoconstrictor [274]. Several of the prostaglandins and leukotrienes released by airway epithelium stimulate ciliary beat frequency [1]. HETEs and EETs generated by both lipoxygenase and cytochrome P450 monooxygenase have multiple effects on airway function [275].

Multiple studies have shown that airway smooth muscle becomes more sensitive to a wide variety of contractile agents when the epithelium is removed. In some cases, this inhibitory action of the epithelium is ascribable to its barrier or metabolic functions, but bioassay and other approaches provide considerable evidence for epithelial-derived inhibitory or relaxing factors (EpDIF or EpDRF). However, the identity of such factors remains elusive, and it seems likely that the relaxant effect of airway epithelium is due mainly to a variable mixture of NO and arachidonic acid metabolites, of which PGE_2 may be the most important [276].

Neuroendocrine cells contain a variety of mediators that are released across the basolateral membrane in response to hypoxia and other stimuli. Serotonin and gastrin-releasing peptide are quantitatively the most important of the released compounds, which may also include calcitonin, calcitonin gene-related peptide, endothelin, leu-enkephalin and somatostatin [89, 90].

Other biologically active compounds secreted by airway surface epithelium include nitric oxide (NO) [230], endothelin [277], glutathione [278] and acetylcholine [279]. NO has multiple actions. It regulates ciliary beat frequency, alters transepithelial ion transport, kills bacteria and viruses, stimulates mucus secretion, promotes wound repair, induces cytokine production, defends against viral infection and promotes apoptosis [230]. There is conflicting evidence for transcytosis of albumin in either the secretory or absorptive direction by airway epithelium [280, 281].

An enzyme, enkephalinase (neutral endopeptidase) that degrades peptides released from sensory nerve terminals is found on the membranes of airway epithelial cells. Inhibition of this enzyme with thiorphan in vitro increases the effects of substance P on gland secretion, smooth muscle contraction, and ciliary beat frequency [282]. There is evidence that levels of epithelial neutral endopeptidase are reduced during inflammation. This would lead to elevated levels of peptides, which will contribute to airway hyperreactivity by actions on sensory nerves and smooth muscle [282]. Airway epithelial cell membranes also contain histamine N-methyltransferase, an enzyme that breaks down histamine [283].

2.7   TRANSPORT OF ACID AND BASE

Airway surface liquid is normally slightly acidic (pH ~6.85) relative to plasma [284]. It becomes more alkaline with chronic bronchitis, pneumonia and colds (up to pH 8.3), and acidifies in cystic fibrosis and asthma (to as low as pH 6.0) [284, 285]. These pathological changes in pH could affect airway defense by altering, among other things, transepithelial salt and water transport, the visco-elastic properties of mucus, and the activity of antimicrobials [285, 286].

What factors determine ASL pH? First, there is the buffer capacity of ASL. Second, there are several routes by which HCO_3^- can enter the ASL. Third, there are at least three mechanisms of H^+ secretion by airway epithelium.

ASL has a buffer capacity (the number of moles of strong acid or base needed to change pH by one unit) of ~14 mM/pH at pH 7.0 [287]. Most of this is attributable to HCO_3^- [288], which enters ASL in two ways. First, it diffuses down a concentration gradient across the tight junctions [289]. Second, it is actively secreted by the epithelium. It is accumulated in the cells either by the actions of carbonic anhydrase or by entry across the basolateral membrane by cotransport with Na^+ [290, 291]. It then diffuses down its electrochemical gradient across the apical membrane through CFTR and possibly other anion channels (see Figure 12).

In fact, in vivo, HCO_3^- rather than Cl^- may be the predominant anion secreted by tracheal epithelium. Thus, under open-circuit conditions, V_a (the apical membrane voltage) of tracheal epithelium is −30 mV [292], $[Cl^-]_i$ is ~ 43 mM [293] and ASL $[Cl^-]$ may be ~120 mM (see Section 2.10). These numbers generate a net electrochemical driving force for Cl^- across the apical membrane of 3 mV directed outwardly. In short, Cl^- is close to equilibrium across the apical membrane, and net Cl^- secretion is close to zero. By contrast, the electrical gradient for HCO_3^- can be calculated as strongly outwards. ASL will be exposed alternately to air on inspiration ($P_{CO2} \approx 0$ mm Hg) and alveolar gases ($P_{CO2} \approx 40$ mm Hg) on expiration, for a time-averaged P_{CO2} of ~20 mm Hg. For an ASL pH of 6.85, this corresponds to a $[HCO_3^-]$ of 3.4 mM. P_{CO2} in cells may be assumed to be an average of that in ASL (20 mm Hg) and arterial blood (40 mm Hg), i. e. ~30 mm Hg. For the recorded pH_i of ~6.95 [294], the corresponding $[HCO_3^-]_i$ is ~6.4 mM. Thus, there is an outwardly directed concentration gradient for HCO_3^- across the apical membrane, which combined with V_a generates a net outwardly directed electrochemical gradient for HCO_3^- of ~47 mV. HCO_3^- is

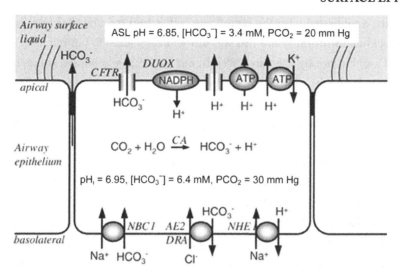

FIGURE 12: Acid–base balance in airway epithelium. The major transport proteins regulating acid/base balance are shown as well as estimates of P_{CO2}, [HCO_3] and pH for ASL and cytoplasm. See text for details.

therefore predicted to be the major secreted anion through CFTR despite the fact that P_{HCO3}/P_{Cl} for CFTR is only ~0.2 [295]. As discussed in the next section, the apical membrane of airway epithelium also contains calcium-activated Cl^- channels (CaCC) and SLC26A9, another anion channel, and there is evidence for HCO_3^- flux through both of these [296, 297].

The values for pH and [HCO_3^-] for the ASL and cell interior are summarized in Figure 12. It must be admitted that the pH_i used was determined in vivo with P_{CO2} of 40 mm Hg. Nevertheless pH_i is likely to be under tight homeostatic control (by HCO_3^-/Cl^- and Na^+/H^+ exchange) and unlikely to vary much with extracellular P_{CO2}. The estimate of [HCO_3^-] for ASL shown in Figure 12 should be viewed cautiously. The range of pH values reported for normal ASL is 6.5 to 7.7 [285]. P_{CO2} in vitro is usually 40 mm Hg. In vivo it probably averages 20 mm Hg. Depending on which values of P_{CO2} and pH are used, the Henderson–Hasselbalch Equation yields a range of [HCO_3^-] from 1.5 to 48 mEq/l!

In addition to the bicarbonate-secreting pathways, three different groups have each identified a different proton transport pathway in the apical membrane of airway epithelium (Figure 12). One group bathed intact distal bronchi of the pig in HCO_3^--buffered saline and perfused their lumens with a HCO_3^--free saline with an initial pH of 7.0 [298]. This perfusate acidified, an effect that was blocked by bafilomycin (an inhibitor of vacuolar H^+–ATPase), but not by DMA (an inhibitor of Na^+/H^+ exchange) [298]. In a second study, physiological saline (100 µl, pH ~7.5) was added to the mucosal surface of primary cultures of human nasal epithelium (1 cm^2 area). Samples were taken at intervals, equilibrated with the same P_{CO2} as the cultures, and their pH determined. The mucosal saline acidified with time, and this was blocked by Sch28080 (an inhibitor of the colonic-type H^+/K^+ATPase) but not by ouabain [289]. In our studies, we mounted sheets of primary cultures of human tracheal epithelium between plastic half-chambers. The serosal face of the sheets was bathed with HCO_3^--buffered medium and the mucosal surface with HCO_3^--free saline (initial pH of 7.3). The rate of proton transfer was then determined by pH-stat [299]. Under basal conditions, the mucosal medium acidified at a rate corresponding to transepithelial proton secretion of ~0.2 μEq cm^{-2} h^{-1} that was increased by either histamine or ATP. In combination, these agents increased H^+ secretion by 3.5-fold. Added after ATP plus histamine, Zn^{2+} (a blocker of proton channels) markedly inhibited proton secretion. Bafilomycin, Sch28080, ouabain or amiloride, however, were without effect. Recently, the proton channels involved have been identified as HVCN1 [300].

Though the ATPases will transport H^+ against its electrochemical gradient, net H^+ secretion via proton channels can only be thermodynamically downhill. For the pH values shown in Figure 12, the net electrochemical gradient for H^+ will be outward for all values of the apical membrane voltage, V_a, more negative than −6 mV. However, the driving force will be increased when inflammatory mediators such as histamine and ATP elevate $[Ca^{2+}]_i$. This is because the apical membrane contains a Ca-activated DUOX-based NADPH oxidase [248] that oxidizes NADPH to NADP$^+$ and H^+ and two electrons. The cytosol is thus acidified, and the cell membrane is depolarized by the outward electron current [301]. Both changes increase the outwardly directed electrochemical gradient for H^+. An appealing feature of this system is the linkage of H^+ secretion to electron secretion—the electrons react with O_2 to produce superoxide that in turn generates hydrogen peroxide and hypochlorous acid, both of which play important roles in airway defense.

In recent studies on H^+ efflux across the apical membrane [288], beads of alkaline saline (pH 7.6) were placed on the surface of pig tracheas and their pH monitored with dextran-BCECF. They acidified in response to a combination of ATP and histamine at a rate that was unaffected by bafilomycin, Sch28080 or ouabain. This provides evidence against colonic or gastric-type H^+/K^+ATPases and vacuolar ATPase. Unfortunately, Zn^{2+} could not be tested as it interfered with the fluorescence measurements.

The relative importance of the three proton-secreting pathways is unclear, but presumably varies with the degree of stimulation of the cells by inflammatory and neurohumoral mediators [299]. Also, airway regions may differ in their proton secreting mechanisms as may cultured and native epithelia. Finally, the method used may influence which transporters are detected. Nevertheless, the discovery of three independent proton-secreting pathways in airway epithelium indicates the importance of regulating ASL pH.

Na^+/H^+ and HCO_3^-/Cl^- exchangers are also present in airway epithelium, but appear to be exclusively basolateral [288, 294, 302] and concerned mainly with intracellular pH regulation.

2.8 ACTIVE ION TRANSPORT

2.8.1 General

The major transepithelial ion transport processes in the airways are active Na^+ absorption and active Cl^- secretion. These are electrogenic; they set up a lumen negative transepithelial potential difference (V_{te}) that in humans in vivo is 30 mV for mucociliary epithelium in the nose, 32 mV in the trachea, 20 mV in large bronchi, and 14 mV in small [303, 304]. Similar values for V_{te} have been described for dog airways [305]. Across species, the in vivo tracheal V_{te} also depends on airway size (Figure 13). So too does short-circuit current (I_{sc}) (Figure 13), which as described next is approximately equal to the sum of active Na^+ absorption and active Cl^- secretion. This dependence of I_{sc} on airway size is to be expected given that epithelial height, and therefore the total amount of cell membrane, increases with airway size. Primary cultures of airway epithelium display a similar dependence of I_{sc} on cell height [306, 307].

A possible factor in the lower V_{te}s of smaller airways is that their epithelia are more prone to damage by the exploring electrode (usually agar or saline in polyethylene tubing of ~1 mm o. d.). However, if one calculates transepithelial electrical resistance, R_{te}, from the values of V_{te} and I_{sc} shown in Figure 1 ($R_{te} = V_{te} / I_{sc}$), the values average ~500 Ω cm^2 and show no dependence on body mass (i. e. tracheal size).

The V_{te} drives passive movement of counterions in the shunt pathways (usually mainly the paracellular pathway) to maintain electroneutrality. In a Na^+-absorbing epithelium, for instance,

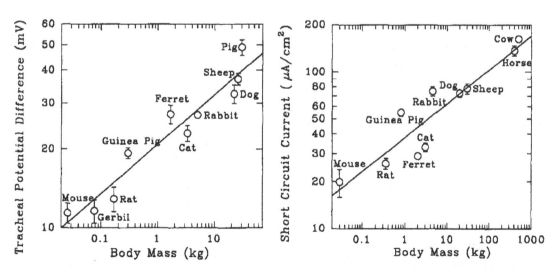

FIGURE 13: Dependence of tracheal electrical properties on body mass. Left panel) Transepithelial voltage measured in vivo. Right panel) Short-circuit current measured in vitro. Taken from ref. [308].

the V_{te} set up by active Na^+ transfer will drive some Na^+ back through the shunt, but will also pull some Cl^- forward. The current in the active pathway equals the current in the passive, but the contribution of the various ions to the current in the active and passive pathways differs, and this is why net salt transfer occurs. For maximum absorption of $NaCl/NaHCO_3$, a Na-absorbing epithelium would have anion selective tight junctions. Similarly, a Cl^--secreting epithelium would need cation-selective tight junctions. The tight junctions in airway epithelium are approximately equally permeable to anions and cations [152] consistent with the comparatively low baseline fluid flows across this epithelium (see p. 20), and with the hypothesis that fluid flows can be finely controlled by altering tight junctional permselectivity [152].

2.8.2 Ussing Chambers

Because of their potential role in regulating ASL depth, the active ion transport processes of airway epithelia have been investigated with Ussing chambers from at least 1968 [309]. In this approach, an epithelial sheet is mounted between half-chambers so as to separate media bathing the mucosal (apical) and serosal (basolateral) surfaces. Current flowing through an external circuit is adjusted to clamp V_{te} to zero. This current is known as the short-circuit current (I_{sc}), and providing certain conditions are met it is equal to the sum of all the active transport processes operating across the tissue [310]. The specific ion transport processes responsible for generating the I_{sc} can be determined from measurement of transepithelial fluxes of radioactive tracers, ion substitution experiments, or the use of specific transport blockers. In airway epithelia, the sum of active Na^+ absorption and active Cl^- secretion is approximately equal to the I_{sc}, suggesting that other active ion transport processes are comparatively minor in magnitude [136, 308].

Table 3 lists the predominant active ion transport processes of airway epithelia, as determined from Ussing chamber studies on short-circuited tissues; full details are provided elsewhere [136, 308]. Under baseline conditions, active absorption of Na^+ predominates across many airway epithelia. In others active secretion of Cl^- is the major ion transport process. A few show approximately equal amounts of both. There is a switch from Cl^- secretion to Na^+ absorption during development. In the fetus, the water flow that accompanies Cl^- secretion provides a turgor pressure that helps the lungs expand and develop [311]. At birth, a switch to Na^+ absorption (in both airway and pulmonary epithelium) removes the liquid and allows the lungs to fill with air [312]. In tracheal epithelium of adult dogs and cattle, active Cl^- secretion may reflect inflammation as it is abolished by indomethacin, the inhibitor of prostaglandin synthesis [271, 313]. In adult human airways Na^+ absorption is the major active ion transport process present under baseline conditions [33, 34, 306, 314], and even when induced by elevation of intracellular Ca^{2+} or cAMP active Cl^- secretion is of small magnitude and transient duration [34, 306].

TABLE 3: Major active ion transport processes of airway epithelia under resting conditions.

Only Cl^- secretion	
Fetal sheep trachea	[315]
Fetal dog trachea	[316]
Newborn dog trachea	[316]
Only Na^+ absorption	
Pig nasal	[309]
Human nasal	[314]
Human trachea	[306]
Human bronchus	[33]
Human bronchiole	[34]
Dog bronchus	[317]
Pig bronchus	[318]
Sheep bronchus	[315]
Sheep trachea	[319]
Sheep distal airway	[320]
Monkey trachea	[318]
Guinea pig trachea	[318]
Rabbit nasal	[321]
Rabbit trachea	[322]

TABLE 3: (*continued*)	
Cl$^-$ secretion and Na$^+$ absorption	
Dog main stem bronchus	[317]
Rabbit trachea	[309]
Ferret trachea	[323]
Cow trachea	[313]
Cat trachea	[323]
Dog trachea	[324]
Horse trachea	[325]
Pig Bronchiole	[35]

2.8.3   Mechanisms of Active Cl$^-$ Secretion and Active Na$^+$ Absorption

Directional transport of ions by epithelia requires the presence of different transport proteins in their apical and basolateral membranes. The apical membrane of airway epithelia contains Na$^+$ and Cl$^-$ channels, but has negligible K$^+$ conductance. The basolateral membrane, however, is K$^+$-selective containing both cAMP- and Ca-activated K channels. The Na$^+$–K$^+$–ATPase and a Na$^+$–K$^+$–2Cl$^-$ cotransporter (NKCC) are also restricted to the basolateral membrane. The way that this polarization of transport proteins brings about active secretion of Cl$^-$ is illustrated in Figure 14. Entry of Cl$^-$ across the basolateral membrane is by cotransport with Na$^+$ (and K$^+$). The energy in the transmembrane concentration gradient for Na$^+$ allows Cl$^-$ to be accumulated within the cells to a level greater than that predicted for passive distribution according to the apical membrane potential difference (V_a) [326]. There is therefore a net exit of Cl$^-$ across this membrane through conductive pathways. The known values of the electrochemical gradient and the Cl$^-$ conductance indicate that this movement need be nothing other than diffusional [292, 327]. The Na$^+$ that enters by cotransport with Cl$^-$ is removed from the cells by basolaterally located Na$^+$–K$^+$–ATPase [328]. The ATPase also pumps in K$^+$, which, together with the K$^+$ entering by NKCC, recycles through the basolateral membrane K$^+$ channels [329].

The mechanism of Na$^+$ absorption across airway epithelia is as first described in 1958 for frog skin [330] (see Figure 14). Sodium ions flow down their electrochemical gradient into the

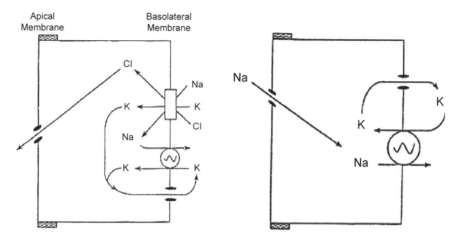

Apical   Basolateral
Membrane   Membrane

FIGURE 14: Cl secretion and Na absorption by airway epithelium. See text for details.

cell through Na^+ channels (epithelial Na^+ channels; ENaC) in the apical membrane. They are then extruded across the basolateral membrane in exchange for K^+ by the Na^+–K^+–ATPase; the K^+ recycles across the basolateral membrane through K^+ channels.

The model for Cl^- secretion has been tested extensively for dog tracheal epithelium [326], and the following discussion refers to this tissue. However, all indications are that the mechanisms of Cl^- secretion by other airway epithelia are identical to those of dog trachea. Under short-circuit conditions in dog tracheal epithelium $V_a = V_b$ (basolateral membrane potential) = –50 to –60 mV. Ion-sensitive microelectrodes show that aNa_i ranges from 10 to 20 mM, aCl_i from 30 to 50 mM, and aK_i from 69 to 83 mM [293, 327, 331, 332], and similar values have been reported for human nasal epithelium [333, 334]. The sum of the transmembrane potential difference and the potential calculated from the Nernst equation give the electrochemical driving force for any particular ion. For the above values, this is outward for Cl^- and K^+, and markedly inward for Na^+.

Basolateral cotransport of Na^+, K^+ and Cl^- is responsible for accumulation of intracellular Cl^- to concentrations greater than predicted for passive distribution according to V_a. Thus, in short-circuited tissues, Welsh [293] measured aCl_i of 38 mM, considerably above the level of 14 mM predicted for passive distribution. Removal of serosal Na^+, however, or inhibition of NKCC with loop diuretics, caused aCl_i to fall to levels not significantly different from those for passive distribution.

The initial evidence for the relative ion selectivities of apical and basolateral membranes came from ion substitution experiments. Changes in the mucosal concentrations of Na^+ and Cl^- (but not of K^+) affected apical membrane potential indicating that it is conductive to Cl^- and Na^+ (but not K^+). By contrast, V_b was affected by changes in serosal K^+ concentration (to the degree predicted by the Nernst equation), but not by changes in serosal Cl^- or Na^+ [292, 329].

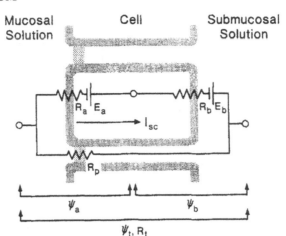

FIGURE 15: Equivalent circuit model for airway epithelium. R_a—apical membrane resistance; E_a—apical membrane electromotive force (emf); R_b and E_a basolateral membrane resistance and emf; R_p—paracellular (shunt) resistance; R_t—transepithelial resistance; ψ_a, ψ_b and ψ_t—apical, basolateral and transepithelial voltages. Taken from ref. [335].

In an Ussing chamber, one can determine transepithelial voltage and resistance (V_{te} and R_{te}) and I_{sc} ($= V_{te}/R_{te}$). If the Ussing chamber is modified to allow a microelectrode to be inserted into the cell, then V_a, V_b and the fractional resistance (f_R) can also be determined. This last is the ratio of R_a to R_{te} determined from the deflections in V_a and V_{te} in response to current pulses across the tissue ($f_R = \Delta V_a/\Delta V_{te} = R_a/R_{te}$). This form of electrophysiological analysis was first performed on airway epithelium by Welsh et al. [292]. They noted that the stimulation of Cl⁻ secretion across dog tracheal epithelium by epinephrine was biphasic. In the first phase, I_{sc} and V_{te} increased, f_R decreased, R_{te} decreased, and V_a and V_b depolarized; all changes consistent with an increase in apical membrane Cl⁻ conductance. In the second phase, I_{sc} and V_{te} continued to increase, but V_a and V_b hyperpolarized, f_R increased and R_{te} continued to decrease. These changes are consistent with an increase in basolateral K⁺ conductance.

By following these parameters over time and assuming that the paracellular resistance (R_p) did not change in response to activation of Cl⁻ secretion, the microelectrode measurements described above were used to model the epithelium as an equivalent circuit [335] (see Figure 15). This analysis showed that E_b was about −80 mV, close to E_K (the Nernst potential for K), and did not change significantly on stimulating Cl⁻ secretion. This is consistent with the only significant conductance in this membrane being to K⁺. By contrast, E_a ranged from E_{Na} to E_{Cl}, depending on the individual tissue and the treatment. In resting tissues treated with indomethacin to abolish baseline Cl⁻ transport, E_a averaged +25 mV (i.e., close to E_{Na}). On stimulation with epinephrine and opening of Cl$^-$ channels E_a became -30 mV (i.e., close to E_{Cl}). The conclusion is that the apical membrane has both a Na$^+$ and Cl$^-$ conductance (G_{Na} and G_{Cl}). Under resting conditions G_{Na} is the greater, under stimulated conditions G_{Cl} predominates.

Similar conclusions were later obtained from equivalent circuit analysis of human nasal epithelium [334, 336] and by a second group working on dog tracheal epithelium [337]. Of particular interest was work on cultured cells derived from nasal epithelium from patients with cystic fibrosis (CF) in which lack of the CFTR-dependent G_{Cl} shifted E_a from -1 to $+43$ mV [336] thereby nicely demonstrating that E_a of non-CF cells reflects a balance between G_{Cl} and G_{Na}.

The apical membrane contains both Na$^+$ and Cl$^-$ channels, and the same cell (presumably the ciliated cell) simultaneously actively absorbs Na$^+$ while actively secreting Cl$^-$ (electroneutrality is maintained because exit, of Cl$^-$ or Na$^+$, on one membrane is matched by entry on the other). This means that there is a reciprocal relationship between Cl$^-$ secretion and Na$^+$ absorption caused by changes in both V_a and intracellular ion content. For instance, blocking ENaC with amiloride inhibits Na$^+$ absorption, and by hyperpolarizing the apical membrane stimulates Cl$^-$ secretion [338]. Increases in Cl$^-$ secretion will tend to inhibit Na$^+$ absorption [271, 339] because opening Cl$^-$ channels will depolarize V_a and activation of NKCC will raise [Na]$_i$.

2.8.4   Under Open-Circuit Conditions Active Secretion of Cl$^-$ Is Reduced or Abolished

The Cl$^-$ secretion seen in short-circuited tissues in Ussing chambers will be reduced or even absent under open-circuit conditions. This is because there is an essentially reciprocal relationship between V_{te} and V_a (see Figure 16). First described for dog tracheal epithelium [292], this relationship was later confirmed for primary cultures of bovine tracheal epithelium [340].

This relationship between V_a and V_{te} applies because V_b is essentially constant over the physiological range of V_{te}. This is readily understandable from the relationship: $V_b = E_b + I_{sc}R_b$. The only important conductance in the basolateral membrane is to K$^+$, so E_b is equal to E_K and constant. Further, alterations in I_{sc} achieved by varying either Cl$^-$ secretion or Na$^+$ absorption will be accompanied by approximately equal but opposite proportional changes in R_b, and the term $I_{sc}R_b$ will also be approximately constant. Thus, V_b changes little with changes in active Na$^+$ absorption or active Cl$^-$ secretion. If V_b is constant, the expression, $V_{te} = V_a + V_b$, shows that changes in V_{te} must result in equal and opposite changes in V_a. The reason that V_a varies with V_{te} can also be appreciated from an inspection of the relationship, $V_a = E_a + I_{sc}R_a$. The term, $I_{sc}R_{te}$, will not vary much with changes in active Cl$^-$ secretion or Na$^+$ absorption. However, changes in Na$^+$ or Cl$^-$ transport will shift E_a between E_{Cl} and E_{Na} depending on the relative values of apical membrane Cl$^-$ and Na$^+$ conductances. V_a will shift by approximately the same amount as E_a, and V_{te} will shift by the same amount in the opposite direction.

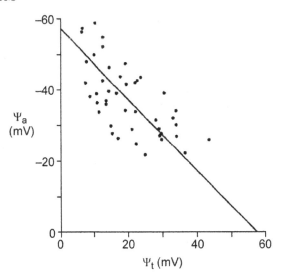

FIGURE 16: Reciprocal relationship between V_a and V_{te} in dog tracheal epithelium. The line has been drawn with a gradient of -1, but is not significantly different from the best least squares regression. Taken from ref. [292].

In short, under open-circuit conditions an increase in V_{te} will depolarize V_a and reduce (or reverse) the driving force for Cl^- exit. In cultures of human nasal epithelium Cl^- has been reported to be in equilibrium across the apical membrane at a V_{te} of -10 mV [334]. As discussed earlier, taking a value of 120 mM [Cl] in ASL [341], and assuming $[Cl]_i$ of 43 mM, then the electrochemical gradient for Cl across the apical membrane is zero when $V_a = -27$ mV. V_b in actively secreting tissues is -55 mV [292], so V_{te} at which Cl is in equilibrium across the apical membrane comes to -28 mV. Measurements of transepithelial fluid flows indicated that the electrochemical gradient for Cl^- across the apical membrane of primary cultures of either human or bovine tracheal epithelium was zero at $\sim\!-35$ mV [340]. Others have estimated V_{te} at which Cl^- is at equilibrium as -42 mV [337].

Thus, for dog and human tracheas, at the in vivo V_{te} of $\sim\!30$ mV Cl^- should be close to equilibrium across the apical membrane, and there will be little or no Cl^- secretion. As airways become smaller, V_{te} decreases, and it is possible that these small airways do show active Cl^- secretion under open-circuit conditions. It is also possible that V_b is less in these small airways, and the V_{te} at which Cl^- becomes passively distributed across the apical membrane is also less. Unfortunately, these small airways have not been studied with microelectrodes.

Even supposing that the electrochemical gradient for Cl^- is outwardly directed across the apical membrane in vivo, stimulation of Cl^- secretion across native human tracheal epithelium by elevation of either cAMP or $[Ca^{2+}]_i$ is transient (see Figure 20D). And the same is true for primary cultures of human bronchiolar epithelium (Figure 17).

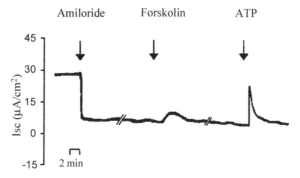

FIGURE 17: Stimulation of Cl⁻ secretion across primary cultures of human bronchiolar epithelium is transient. In the presence of amiloride, I_{sc} is thought to reflect predominantly active Cl⁻ secretion. Taken from ref. [34].

2.8.5   Coordination of Transporter Activities

In epithelia, the turnover rates for the intracellular pools of transported ions are in the order of seconds or minutes [342]. In tracheal epithelium, for instance, a Cl-dependent I_{sc} of 100 μA/cm^2 means that net influx of Cl⁻ across the basolateral membrane is 4 μEq cm^{-2} h^{-1}. For a cell height of 50 μm and an aCl$_i$ of 38 mM, this would result in doubling of aCl$_i$ within ~30 sec. Thus, when the rate of net Cl⁻ secretion increases, to avoid problems with intracellular osmolarity and volume control, it is important that the turnover rates of all the transport proteins involved change in parallel [342]. In the dog trachea, studies by Welsh, Frizzell and others [292, 332, 335], suggest the following sequence of events: an initial increase in apical membrane G_{Cl} somehow causes basolateral NKCC to turn over faster (which it must if Cl⁻ secretion is going to be maintained). This brings more Na$^+$ into the cell, elevating [Na$^+$]$_i$, and stimulating the Na$^+$-K$^+$–ATPase, thereby increasing influx of K$^+$ across the basolateral membrane. Basolateral G_K now increases, serving two functions. First, by current flow in the tissue's shunt pathways, the increase in G_K hyperpolarizes the apical membrane, thereby retaining the driving force for net Cl⁻ exit across this membrane (an increase in G_{Cl} alone will depolarize the membrane and the increase in Cl⁻ conductance will be offset by a decrease in the driving force for Cl⁻ exit). Second, the increased G_K allows the increased amounts of K$^+$ entering by the NKCC and the Na$^+$–K$^+$–ATPase to recycle across the basolateral membrane, thereby avoiding problems of volume control. In fact, on induction of Cl⁻ secretion, increases in turnover of the different transport proteins involved are so well matched that changes in intracellular ion contents on induction of Cl⁻ secretion are quite small. Thus, in dog tracheal epithelium, aCl$_i$ shifts from 47 to 32 mM, aNa$_i$ from 11 to 21 mM, and aK$_i$ from 83 to 69 mM [327, 331, 332].

During changes in Cl⁻ secretion, how exactly are the turnover rates of the various transporters coordinated in the absence of marked changes in the driving forces for the various ions? Some of the matching is undoubtedly due to the fact that the transporters respond to the same second messengers. For instance, there are separate Cl^- channels in the apical membrane that respond to either Ca^{2+} or cAMP, and the same is true of K^+ channels in the basolateral membrane. The NKCC can be activated by cAMP but apparently not Ca^{2+} [343]. During Ca-induced Cl^- secretion coupling between Cl^- exit via apical G_{Cl} and Cl^- entry via basolateral NKCC is probably mediated by a Cl^--sensing protein kinase. Opening of Cl^- channels in the apical membrane causes an initial drop in $[Cl^-]_i$ that activates the kinase leading to increased phosphorylation and turnover of the NKCC [344]. The increased influx of Na^+ on the NKCC will elevate $[Na^+]_i$ and stimulate the Na^+-K^+-ATPase so that pumped efflux of Na^+ matches the increased influx. At normal levels of $[Na^+]_i$, the relation between Na^+-K^+-ATPase activity and $[Na^+]_i$ is very steep [345], and the necessary increase in Na^+-K^+-ATPase activity is achieved with only a small change in $[Na^+]_i$ [331]. There is no relationship between G_K and either V_b or NaKATPase activity [346], so presumably the K^+ channels are opened sufficiently by the same second messengers that open the apical membrane Cl^- channels.

There is evidence that Ca^{2+} elevates cAMP and vice versa. In airway serous gland acini, elevation of cAMP elevates $[Ca^{2+}]_i$ sufficiently to activate basolateral G_K, but not CaCC [65]. It is not known whether this occurs in surface epithelium, but isoproterenol does elevate $[Ca^{2+}]_i$ in primary cultures of human tracheal epithelium, and the isoproterenol-induced increase in I_{sc} exactly parallels the change in $[Ca^{2+}]_i$ [347]. As discussed in the next section, the converse occurs: elevation of $[Ca^{2+}]_i$ stimulates a Ca-dependent adenylate cyclase, elevating cAMP and activating CFTR [348].

2.8.6 Apical Membrane Cl Conductance

Primary cultures of human tracheal epithelium showed increases in amiloride-insensitive I_{sc} when treated with agents that elevate cAMP; these increases were not seen in cultures from patients with cystic fibrosis (Figure 18A). Replacing Cl^- in the mucosal medium with a large impermeant anion resulted in depolarization of V_a in non-CF cultures, but a slight hyperpolarization in CF cultures (Figure 18B). Thus, in CF, the epithelium seems to be lacking a cAMP-mediated Cl^- conductance.

This was later identified as the cystic fibrosis transmembrane conductance regulator, a cAMP-activated Cl^- channel. Loss-of-function mutations in the gene for this channel cause cystic fibrosis, and an abundance of evidence suggested that this was the predominant apical membrane Cl^- channel mediating cAMP-dependent Cl secretion [350]. For instance, whole-cell patch-clamping showed cAMP-activated currents with the biophysical signature of this channel, specific blockers of this channel inhibit cAMP-induced Cl^- currents in Ussing chambers and patches, and CFTR is localized to the apical membrane of ciliated cells (Figure 19). It was known that Cl^- secretion could

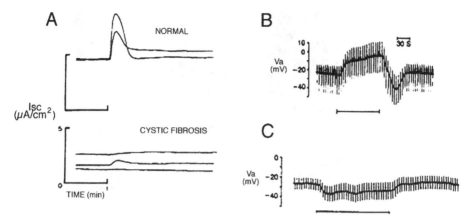

FIGURE 18: Lack of Cl⁻ secretion and apical membrane Cl⁻ conductance in human tracheal epithelium in CF. A) Added at 1 min, isoproterenol stimulated I_{sc} in non-CF but not CF cells. B) Replacing Cl⁻ in the mucosal medium with gluconate (horizontal bar) caused a depolarization of V_a in non-CF cells. C) The same maneuver caused a small hyperpolarization of V_a in CF cells. Taken from ref. [349].

be stimulated by agents that elevated intracellular Ca^{2+}. But this could be explained by activation of basolateral K^+ channels [351], hyperpolarization of the apical membrane and an increase in the driving force for Cl⁻ exit through constitutively open CFTR. However, it is now known that at least two other Cl⁻ channels are present in the apical membrane of airway epithelia: calcium-activated Cl channels (CaCC) and the constitutively active SLC26A9.

CaCC are ubiquitous in the membranes of epithelia and other cells, and often respond directly to Ca^{2+} rather than to Ca-dependent phosphorylation [352]. The first indication of apical membrane Cl⁻ channels other than CFTR in airway epithelia was that the Ca ionophore, A23187, stimulated amiloride-insensitive I_{sc} to the same degree across primary cultures of both CF and non-CF human tracheal epithelium [353]. Microelectrode studies provided more direct evidence for Ca-dependent activation of apical membrane Cl⁻ channels in human airway epithelium. Thus, A23187 (and also ionomycin) caused a drop in $R_a / (R_a + R_b)$. Further, if A23187 was added with low Cl⁻ in the mucosal medium (3 mM), then there was a significant drop in aCl$_i$ [334]. However, the most direct evidence for CaCC came from preparations in which the basolateral membrane had been permeabilized with nystatin and a Cl⁻ concentration gradient imposed across the apical membrane [354]. Addition of Ca ionophore caused transient increases in Cl⁻ current across these preparations, whereas cAMP caused a sustained increase. The cAMP-induced response was missing in CF cells but the Ca-dependent response was unchanged (Figure 20A).

In Ussing chambers, primary cultures of human tracheal epithelium showed transient increases in I_{sc} in response to a number of Ca-elevating agents that in their time courses exactly

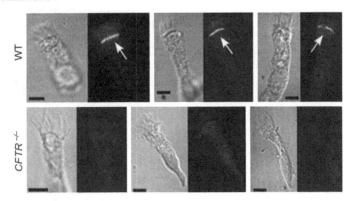

FIGURE 19: CFTR localizes to the apical membrane of ciliated cells from non-CF pig tracheal epithelium, but is undetectable in cells from the CF transgenic pig. Pictures are paired DIC images and immunocytochemical staining for CFTR (arrows). Scale bars = 5 μm. Taken from ref. [65].

paralleled changes in $[Ca^{2+}]_i$. Interestingly, this was also true of isoproterenol, an agent that acts predominantly through cAMP (Figure 20B). In later studies, cultures, grown by a different method (Finkbeiner, personal communication), showed both a transient and a sustained increase in I_{sc} to the Ca-elevating agent, UTP (Figure 20C). Use of specific blockers showed that, though CaCC mediated the transient increase, Cl⁻ current during the sustained increase was divided approximately equally through CFTR and CaCC (Figure 20C). It was shown that elevation of cAMP increased $[Ca^{2+}]_i$. This then activated a phosphodiesterase in the same microdomain as CFTR, and the resulting increase in cAMP opened CFTR. Which of these results most closely resembles the situation in native tissue: transient increases in Cl⁻ secretion driven directly by Ca^{2+}, or sustained increases driven largely by Ca-dependent increases in cAMP? I know of only one Ussing chamber record from native human airway epithelium (Figure 20D). The tissue used was a surgical specimen with a reasonable R_{te} of 170 Ω cm² and a high baseline I_{sc} of ~40 μA/cm². However, both isoproterenol and bradykinin induced only transient increases in I_{sc}. The former acts through cAMP, the latter through Ca^{2+} [355]. Amiloride abolished I_{sc}. Similar results, with poorer time resolution, had earlier been obtained on resected human bronchi [33]. Thus, at least in Ussing chambers, there is little baseline Cl⁻ secretion across native human tracheal epithelium, and both Ca^{2+}- and cAMP-dependent increases are of small magnitude and short duration.

In 2008, three research groups identified TMEM16a as possibly accounting for most reports of CaCC activity [356–358]. TMEM16a has been demonstrated in the apical membrane of airway epithelia by immunocytochemistry [359], and use of TMEM16a knock-out animals has strongly implicated this protein as underlying most of the CaCC activity induced by UTP, ATP or cholinergic agents in newborn mouse airway epithelium [360]. In primary cultures of human

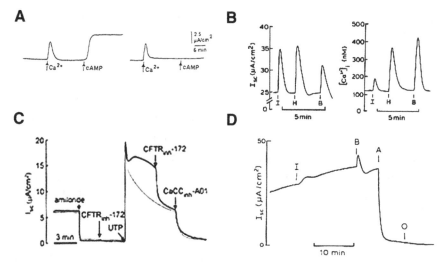

FIGURE 20: Ca-activated Cl⁻ channels in airway epithelia. A) In primary cultures of human tracheal epithelium elevation of cAMP induced Cl⁻ currents across the apical membrane of non-CF cells (left), but not CF (right). Ca-induced currents, however, were unaltered in CF. Taken from ref. [354]. B) In primary cultures of human airway epithelium transient increases in I_{sc} in response to a variety of mediators paralleled changes in $[Ca^{2+}]_i$. I—isoproterenol, H—histamine, B—bradykinin. Taken from ref. [347]. C) In other experiments, elevation of $[Ca^{2+}]_i$ with UTP caused sustained increases in amiloride-insensitive I_{sc} that were inhibited by blockers of either CFTR or CaCC. One tissue received CFTR inhibitor before UTP, the other after. Taken from ref. [348]. E) In native human tracheal epithelium, isoproterenol (I) or bradykinin (B) caused only small transient increases in I_{sc}. A—amiloride, O—ouabain. Taken from ref. [306].

tracheal epithelium, UTP induced transient increases in I_{sc} that were inhibited 50–60% by pretreatment with siRNA against TMEM16a [357]. In a second study with primary cultures of human tracheal epithelium, CF cells were used to avoid the confounding issue of Ca-dependent elevation of cAMP and activation of CFTR (see above). These cells showed both a transient and a sustained increase in I_{sc} in response to UTP. A specific blocker of TMEM16a inhibited the transient increase by ~60% but the sustained increase by only ~15%. By contrast, the same blocker inhibited all the Ca-dependent I_{sc} in salivary gland epithelium [361]. Apparently, under some circumstances, Cl⁻ channels other than TMEM16a may contribute significantly to CaCC-mediated currents in airway epithelium.

Members of the SLC26a family are often Cl⁻/HCO₃⁻ exchangers [362]. However, SCL26A9 is a highly selective Cl⁻ channel [363] expressed at high levels in airway epithelium [364]. A recent study suggests that it is responsible for constitutive Cl⁻ secretion in primary cultures of human airway epithelium and that its activity is dependent on the presence of functional CFTR in the membrane [365].

2.8.7 Epithelial Na⁺ Channel (ENaC)

Amiloride is a highly specific blocker of the epithelial sodium channel (ENaC) [366]. At concentrations that are unlikely to inhibit other transporters, mucosal amiloride reduces I_{sc} across virtually all of a large number of airway epithelia on which it has been tested [326].

Three subunits (α, β, γ) of ENaC have been known for some time. Expression of all three in Xenopus oocytes results in Na currents many-fold larger than when individual subunits, α plus β subunits, or α plus γ subunits are expressed [367]. Recently, atomic force microscopy has shown that most channels assemble as heterotrimers containing one copy of each subunit [368]. It is thought that the α subunit may be essential in bringing the β and γ subunits to the membrane, while the latter two may stabilize the trimer in the membrane. However, individual subunits may also assemble as homotrimers. Thus, in intact polarized alveolar epithelium patch-clamp studies indicate the presence of both $\alpha\beta\gamma$ trimers ($G = \sim8$ pS) and α homomers ($G = \sim25$ pS) [369].

The distribution of the mRNA for the ENaC subunits in the airways has been investigated several times. In human bronchial epithelium, Northern blotting and ISH studies suggested that the relative abundance of mRNA for the three subunits was $\alpha > \beta > \gamma$ [370]. In rat airways, there is some variation along the tracheobronchial tree, and some disagreement between investigators, but as in human bronchus the α-subunit is the commonest [371, 372]. The physiological significance of mRNA for the α-subunit being more abundant than that for the β- and γ-subunits is unclear. Possibly, there is a significant contribution of α-subunit homotrimers to active Na⁺ absorption across the airway epithelium, as in the alveolar.

More recently, a δ subunit has been discovered and shown to function as a Na⁺ channel when combined in trimeric form with β- and γ-subunits [373]. This subunit has been detected in human nasal epithelium, at similar levels to the α subunit, and $\sim50\%$ of the total Na current across the apical membrane has been estimated as being through $\delta\beta\gamma$ trimers rather than $\alpha\beta\gamma$ trimers [374].

Very recently, immunocytochemistry has localized ENaC in human airways to the cilia; it is absent from the apical membrane between the cilia [68].

To conduct Na⁺, segments of the α and γ-subunits of ENaC must be cleaved. This is done by furin-like proteases during ENaC's trafficking to the apical membrane, by extracellular serine proteases, so-called channel-activating proteases (CAPs), once it is in the membrane, or by soluble proteases such as trypsin and neutrophil elastase [375]. Of the CAPs, perhaps the most important is prostasin, which is tethered to the apical membrane by a glycosylphosphatidylinositol (GPI)

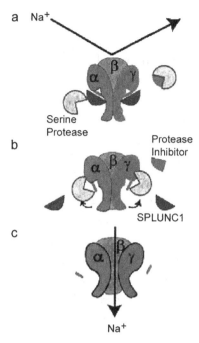

FIGURE 21: Factors regulating ENaC activity. Activation requires cleavage of domains from the α- and γ-subunits by serine (or other) proteases. This cleavage is prevented by SPLUNC. Soluble protease inhibitors also prevent cleavage. Taken from ref. [375].

anchor. Prostasin can be released from the membrane by GPI-specific phospholipase C, or it can be secreted directly. Thus, the degree of activation of ENaC may depend on the balance between membrane-bound and free prostasin in the ASL [375]. In addition, the airway epithelium secretes protease inhibitors into the ASL, of which protease nexin-1 (Pn-1) is best characterized [376]. Finally, SPLUNC1 binds to ENaC and prevents its activation by proteolysis, in part by increasing its endocytosis. These various regulatory influences are summarized in Figure 21. Changes in their balance will influence ENaC activity, thereby potentially influencing the depth of the ASL and promoting mucus accumulation in cystic fibrosis (see Section 4.4.5).

In the airways, cAMP inhibits ENaC when CFTR is present, but stimulates ENaC when CFTR is absent. A drop in aCl_i lowers its activity. Finally, ENaC is not directly sensitive to Ca^{2+}, but is activated by anionic lipids such as PIP_2 and PIP_3 [375]. ENaC in the airways differs from that in other tissues by its insensitivity to aldosterone (probably due to relative lack of receptors), and its activation by glucocorticoids [377], hormones that are important in the stimulation of lung liquid absorption at birth [312].

2.8.8 Basolateral K$^+$ Channels

By 2009, forty-four different types of K channels had been described from alveolar and airway epithelial cells or cell lines [378]. Only two channels, Kv7.1, KCa3.1, have been established as functional in the basolateral membrane of airway epithelium, though there is some evidence that other members of the Kv7 family may be involved.

Kv7.1(also known as KvLQT1), the product of the KCNQ1 gene, has six transmembrane domains and is voltage-sensitive. It has a low conductance (<3 pS) and is activated by cAMP. Use of blockers suggests that it accounts for ~25% of baseline and most of the forskolin-induced increase in Cl$^-$ secretion across airway epithelium [379, 380]. There is pharmacological evidence for the involvement of other channels of the Kv7 family [381]. Immunocytochemistry demonstrated Kv7.1 in basolateral membrane of human tracheal epithelial cultures; Kv7.3 and Kv7.5 were undetectable [381].

KCa3.1 (also known as SH4), the product of the KCNN4 gene, has six-transmembrane-domains and is activated by Ca^{2+}. In nasal epithelium, clotrimazol, a specific blocker of this channel, completely blocks the UTP-dependent increase in I_{sc}, suggesting that this is the major K$^+$ conductance involved in Ca-dependent Cl$^-$ secretion [382]. Further, 1-EBIO, an activator of this channel is a potent stimulator of clotrimazol-sensitive Cl$^-$ secretion across primary cultures of human tracheal epithelium [381].

Patch-clamping studies suggested that BKCa ("Big K—Calcium"), a large conductance (~200 pS), seven trans-membrane-domain Ca-activated K$^+$ channel, is present in the basolateral membrane of human airway epithelial cultures [383]. However, in a recent study the apical membrane of confluent cell sheets of human airway epithelium was permeabilized and a K$^+$ gradient imposed across the tissue. ATP dramatically increased I_{sc} across the preparation, but this was unaffected by blockers of BKCa [384]. It is possible that the patch-clamping studies mis-localized the channel; the assumption that BKCa was in the basolateral membrane was based solely on the finding that K$^+$ channels and Cl$^-$ channels were never observed in the same patch [383].

2.8.9 Na$^+$–K$^+$–2Cl$^-$ Cotransport (NKCC)

Loop diuretics (e.g. bumetanide and furosemide), classical blockers of NaCl cotransport and NKCC, inhibit Cl$^-$ secretion across airway epithelium [326]. Loop diuretics, or removal of serosal Na$^+$, also reduce the aCl$_i$ from a value higher than to the value expected from passive distribution according to V_a [293]. Several early studies showed that this Na$^+$-dependent accumulation of Cl$^-$ by airway epithelium was due to NKCC rather than NaCl cotransport [385, 386].

A series of studies by Haas and co-workers demonstrated that either cAMP or a drop in aCl$_i$ could increase NKCC activity in dog tracheal epithelium [343, 344, 387, 388]. In the first study, [^{3}H]-bumetanide binding to isolated plasma membranes and intact tissues showed that isoproterenol-induced increases in Cl⁻ secretion involved an increase in the numbers of NKCC in the basolateral membrane [387]. Next it was shown that the numbers of transporters was increased by either isoproterenol (cAMP) or UTP (Ca²⁺). The UTP-mediated increase was completely abolished when Cl⁻ efflux across the apical membrane was prevented. However, blocking Cl⁻ efflux inhibited the isoproterenol-induced increase by only ~50% in dog trachea and not at all in human nasal cells. It was concluded that both Ca²⁺ and cAMP stimulate NKCC activity by decreasing aCl_i. In addition, cAMP, but not Ca²⁺, had a direct stimulatory action on transporter numbers. In support of this conclusion, it was shown that a membrane-permeable cAMP analogue increased [³H]-bumetanide binding to CF cells, though clearly in this case there could be no cAMP-dependent Cl⁻ efflux [343]. The dependence of NKCC activity on aCl_i was studied in more detail in cells in which the apical membrane had been permeabilized; the aCl_i of these cells is identical to the aCl_i of the mucosal bathing medium. NKCC activity, measured as the bumetanide-sensitive flux of ³⁶Cl from the serosal to the mucosal side, was shown to increase with decreasing aCl_i [388] (Figure 22A). The final study showed that the bumetanide-sensitive flux was directly proportional to the degree of phosphorylation of NKCC (Figure 22B). A candidate for the Cl-sensing protein kinase has been identified [389].

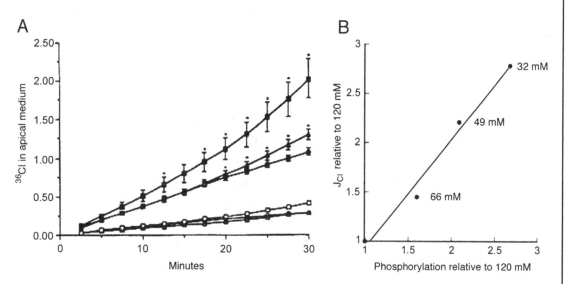

FIGURE 22: Dependence of NKCC activity on aCl_i. A) ³⁶Cl⁻ fluxes across dog tracheal epithelium in which the basolateral membrane had been permeabilized with nystatin. *Squares*—32 mM Cl⁻ in serosal (i.e., intracellular) medium; *triangles*—49 mM Cl⁻; *circles*—66 mM Cl⁻. Open symbols in the presence of bumetanide; closed symbols in the absence. Taken from ref. [388]. B) Correlation between bumetanide-sensitive ³⁶Cl flux and phosphorylation of NKCC. Points represent mean values for the 3 different intracellular Cl concentrations. Data from ref. [344].

Shorofsky et al. [327] have shown that epinephrine increases net Cl⁻secretion across dog tracheal epithelium by ~5 µEq cm^{-2} h^{-1}, and this is associated with a drop in [Cl]$_i$ of ~20 mEq/l. However, the data of Haas et al. (Figure 22) predict a much lower dependence of NKCC activity on aCl$_i$ than this. Two possible factors might resolve this discrepancy. First, epinephrine acts predominantly through cAMP, and this has a direct action on NKCC activity. Second, Haas' experiments were done with aNa$_i$ of ~150 mM, whereas aNa$_i$ in intact cells is ~10 mM, and elevating aNa$_i$ inhibits NKCC [390].

In primary cultures of human airway epithelium and in Calu-3 cells, Liedtke and colleagues [391–393] have shown that hypertonic shock or α_1-adrenergic stimulation activates NKCC by a mechanism involving PKCδ and SPAK (Ste20-related proline alanine-rich kinase). Via linkages to actin these kinases are held in the same microdomain as NKCC, as also is PP2A (protein phosphatase 2A) that opposes the stimulatory effects of the kinases [394].

2.8.10 Na$^+$–K$^+$–ATPase

In airway epithelium, the Na$^+$–K$^+$–ATPase is localized exclusively to the basolateral membrane [328]. Basal, ciliated and goblet cells of airway epithelium all have the same pump density of ~1000 per µm^2 [395]. This is considerably higher than for most non-epithelial cells, and the similarity across airway epithelial cell types suggests that the epithelium functions as a syncytium in which ions readily exchange between cells via gap junctions.

2.8.11 Basolateral Cl⁻ Channels

A number of basolateral Cl⁻ channels have been identified [340, 396–398]. Usually, these are quiescent, and there is no good evidence that they play a role in Cl⁻ secretion. However, they may be involved in cAMP-dependent liquid absorption. Thus, in cell sheets in which V_{te} was more negative than ~30 mV, elevation of intracellular cAMP increased transepithelial liquid absorption [340]. Further, this was blocked by CFTR inhibitors showing that it was driven by the opening of a transcellular route for Cl⁻; active Na$^+$ absorption was unaltered [340]. One of the basolateral Cl⁻ channels was shown to be cAMP-activated. Another was swelling-induced. Therefore, either cAMP opened channels in both membranes or the influx of Cl⁻ consequent on opening of apical membrane CFTR resulted in cell swelling and activation of the swelling-dependent basolateral Cl⁻ channels.

2.8.12 Neurohumoral Regulation

Chloride secretion can be stimulated by virtually anything that elevates intracellular cAMP or Ca^{2+}. Reasonably complete lists of the many chloride secretagogues have been given elsewhere

[136, 326, 399]. Some of the more physiologically relevant of these that act through cAMP include β-adrenergic agents, VIP, PGE_2, CGRP and adenosine [400–404]. The last acts on apical membrane receptors [400]; the others on basolateral. Histamine and ATP (or UTP) act through Ca^{2+} [398, 405, 406]. Both compounds have receptors on both membranes [407–409]. Bradykinin stimulates both directly by raising $[Ca^{2+}]_i$ and indirectly by releasing PGE_2 [355, 410]; it acts predominantly from the mucosal side. Lekotrienes C_4 and D_4 stimulate Cl^- secretion across dog tracheal epithelium secondarily to prostaglandin release [272]. Substance P and neurokinins stimulate Cl^- secretion; the former mainly via Ca^{2+}, the latter via cAMP [411, 412]. Surprisingly, cholinergic agents have little effect on Cl^- secretion across airway epithelia [404, 413, 414]. Menthol is interesting; though most of the Ca-dependent mediators cause large transient increases in $[Ca^{2+}]_i$, menthol causes a small sustained increase associated with a sustained stimulation of Cl^- secretion [415].

Responses to elevation of cAMP tend to be sustained. However, increases in Cl^- secretion in response to elevation of Ca^{2+} are often transient, and caused by direct effects of Ca^{2+} as opposed to Ca-dependent phosphorylation [347, 416]. In human airway epithelium, the time courses of Cl^- secretory responses to a number of agents exactly parallel increases in $[Ca^{2+}]_i$ (see Figure 20B).

Na^+ absorption by airway epithelia is not as markedly affected by cAMP as Cl^- secretion. As discussed earlier, many cAMP-dependent Cl^- secretagogues slightly inhibit active Na^+ absorption by effects on the driving forces for Na^+ entry through ENaC. Accordingly, to test for direct effects of neurohumoral agents on Na^+ absorption, Cullen & Welsh replaced Cl^- in the bathing medium with an impermeant organic anion. Under these circumstances, a variety of cAMP-elevating agents increased I_{sc} (i.e., active Na^+ absorption) by ~25% [417].

Elevation of intracellular Ca^{2+} can profoundly inhibit active Na^+ absorption. Thus, in primary cultures of human tracheal epithelium, the Ca-elevating agent, UTP, first increased (by ~25%) and then inhibited active Na^+ absorption (by ~75%), an effect that was ascribed to down regulation of basolateral K^+ channels [418]. Similar effects have been described for pig tracheal epithelium [419]. Histamine and acetylcholine potently inhibit Na^+ absorption across horse and sheep tracheal epithelia, respectively [407, 414].

2.8.13 Regulation by Intracellular Second Messengers

Beta-adrenergic agents and VIP act via cAMP and stimulate Cl^- secretion when added to the basolateral side of dog tracheal epithelium, but not when added to the apical [403, 404]. Furthermore, their receptors are predominantly basolateral [420, 421]. These mediators presumably use a basolateral adenylate cyclase to generate cAMP, which then diffuses across the cell to activate CFTR.

Adenosine, however, is a cAMP-dependent agonist that acts predominantly on receptors in the apical membrane [400], and this membrane contains all the necessary equipment to regulate cAMP in the immediate vicinity of CFTR. Thus, at least two adenylate cyclases locate to this membrane [348]. Further, at least in Calu-3 cells, PKAII (membrane-bound protein kinase A) is anchored immediately adjacent to CFTR by AKAPs (A kinase anchoring proteins) [266]. In addition, PDE4 (phosphodiesterase E4) is localized in the apical membrane close to CFTR, and provides a diffusion barrier limiting spread of cAMP away from this region [422].

Ca^{2+} elevation by neurohumoral mediators is by the classical phospholipase C pathway that generates IP_3 and DAG from PIP_2. The IP_3 then releases Ca^{2+} from intracellular stores, while the DAG activates protein kinase C (PKC). Activation of PKC stimulates Cl^- secretion across dog tracheal epithelium [423]. With increases in $[Ca^{2+}]_i$ blocked by BAPTA-AM, human nasal cultures still show increases in Cl^- secretion in response to ATP/UTP [424]. These are not seen in CF cells, indicating that they are mediated by CFTR. They are blocked by the PKC inhibitor, chelerythrine [424].

Experiments by Paradiso et al. [425] show that in human airway epithelium Ca^{2+} stores under the apical membrane are functionally separate from those under the basolateral membrane. Sheets of human nasal epithelium were perfused on both sides in Ca^{2+}-free medium to prevent repletion of intracellular Ca^{2+} stores. The cells were then exposed briefly to serosal ATP, serosal ATP again and then mucosal ATP. The first treatment with serosal ATP caused a transient increase in $[Ca^{2+}]_i$, but the second had no effect. The mucosal ATP increased $[Ca^{2+}]_i$. The sequence mucosal ATP/mucosal ATP/serosal ATP likewise led to increase/no effect/increase. Furthermore the increase in $[Ca^{2+}]_i$ in response to mucosal ATP was uninfluenced by prior treatment with serosal ATP and vice versa. Thus, mucosal ATP releases Ca^{2+} from stores under the apical membrane but has no effect on basolateral Ca^{2+} stores. Similarly, activation of basolateral purinergic receptors releases Ca^{2+} from basolateral, but not apical, Ca^{2+} stores. It was also shown that apical stores were recharged entirely from Ca^{2+} entering across the apical membrane, whereas basolateral stores were recharged by Ca^{2+} entering across the basolateral membrane.

As in other epithelia, mitochondria provide the barriers separating these discrete stores. Found in close association with the ER Ca^{2+} stores, they avidly take up Ca^{2+} and limit diffusion of Ca^{2+} through the cell. Following mucosal ATP, apical mitochondria took up Ca^{2+}, basolateral did not. Conversely, serosal UTP increased the Ca^{2+} content of basolateral, but not apical, mitochondria. Addition of basolateral UTP normally has little or no effect on apical membrane CaCC, but is stimulatory when Ca uptake by mitochondria is blocked [426].

2.8.14 K^+ Secretion

Radiotracer studies on short-circuited sheets of airway epithelium have revealed a small component of active K^+ secretion, though this never accounts for more than ~5% of baseline I_{sc} [315, 317, 329]. Further evidence for active K^+ secretion has been obtained with fluorescent K^+-sensing dyes added to the ASL over primary cultures of human tracheal epithelium. The K^+ concentration in the ASL was found to be ~20 mM, considerably higher than the value of 6.5 mM expected for passive distribution according to the V_{te} of 7 mV [381]. Similar values for $[K^+]_{ASL}$ of equine trachea have been obtained with ion-selective microelectrodes [427].

Active K^+ secretion will occur whenever there is a K^+ conductance in the apical membrane. Under baseline conditions, net K^+ secretion across short-circuited airway epithelia averages ~0.05 μEq cm^{-2} h^{-1} [136]. By contrast, across airway epithelia of different species and airway generations, the combination of active Cl^- secretion and active Na^+ absorption generates an I_{sc} of ~3 μEq cm^{-2} h^{-1} [136]. The Na^+–K^+–ATPase is electrogenic, exchanging $2Na^+$ for every $3K^+$. Therefore in a Na^+-absorbing tissue the basolateral K^+ current through K^+ channels is two thirds the Na^+ current across the apical membrane [356]. In a Cl^--secreting epithelium it is 5/6 ths the apical Cl^-current [386]. Accordingly, basolateral K^+ current will be between 2 and 2.5 μEq cm^{-2} h^{-1}. Thus, the K^+ conductance of the apical membrane is only ~2% that of the basolateral [(0.05/2.25) × 100)].

From the changes in V_a, V_t and fR_a, it was concluded that mucosal ATP stimulated active secretion of K^+ across primary cultures of human nasal epithelium [428]. Secretion reached a peak ~30 s after adding ATP, and returned to baseline after ~2 min. In short-circuited tissues, net transepithelial secretion of $^{42}K^+$ was 0.05 μEq cm^{-2} h^{-1} when averaged over the 10-min period after adding ATP.

More recent investigations [384] have confirmed the transient stimulation of K^+ secretion by ATP or UTP. The basolateral membrane of confluent cell sheets of human airway epithelium was permeabilized and a K^+ gradient imposed across the apical membrane. Addition of ATP or UTP induced a large I_{sc} (Figure 23A), which was abolished or markedly inhibited by paxilline or iberiotoxin, blockers of BKCa (Figure 23B and C). In the studies illustrated in Figure 23, forskolin failed to induce K^+ currents across the apical membrane. However, others, using essentially the same preparation, did see a small forskolin-induced increase in K^+ current [381]. This was inhibited by XE991, a broad-spectrum inhibitor of Kv7 channels. Consistent with this, Kv7.1, Kv7.3 and Kv7.5 were demonstrated in the apical membrane by immunocytochemistry [381].

Model simulations indicate that, by hyperpolarizing V_a, activation of an apical membrane K^+ conductance can potentiate the stimulation of Cl^- secretion by UTP or ATP by approximately two-fold [384].

2.8.15 SCN$^-$ Transport

The airway epithelium secretes SCN$^-$ by a mechanism involving uptake across the basolateral membrane on the Na^+/I^- cotransporter followed by efflux across the apical membrane via a variety of pathways including CFTR [429, 430]. The end result is that the concentration of SCN$^-$ in ASL, 0.4 mM, is between ten and a hundred times higher than that in plasma [431]. In the lumen,

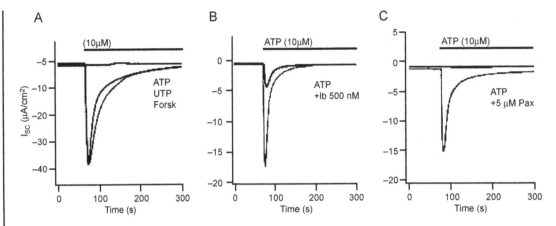

FIGURE 23: BKCa is a Ca-activated apical membrane K^+ channel in airway epithelia. Panels show K^+ currents across human airway epithelial cultures in which the basolateral membrane had been permeabilized. A) Stimulation of currents by ATP and UTP but not forskolin. B & C) Block of ATP-generated currents by blockers of BKCa. Ib—iberiotoxin; Pax—paxilline. Taken from ref. [384].

SCN^- reacts with H_2O_2, generated by DUOX, to form HOSCN that kills bacteria by oxidizing sulfhydryl groups [249]. This reaction is catalyzed by lactoperoxidase secreted by both goblet cells and submucosal glands [223]. In addition to its role as an antimicrobial agent, SCN^- can react with HOCl to form HOSCN and Cl^- [432]. Hypothiocyanate is less toxic to mammalian cells than OCl^- and therefore SCN^- serves a protective function during periods of excess HOCl production by neutrophils.

The Na^+/I^- cotransporter has an affinity for I^- three times that for SCN^-, but the serum I^- concentration is normally 200 to 2000 times less than that of SCN^-. Thus, the concentration of I^- in ASL is undetectable (<0.25 μM). However, ingesting a standard KI pill (of the kind used to prevent thyroid damage after exposure to radioactive iodide isotopes) will increase plasma I^- to 500 μM, about the same as the SCN^- concentration. Under these conditions, sufficient hypoiodous acid (HOI) is produced by LPO-catalyzed reaction with H_2O_2 to have significant antiviral actions [433].

2.8.16 Ca^{2+} Transport

As determined from transepithelial fluxes of ^{45}Ca, under short-circuit conditions there is a significant net Ca^{2+} secretion of ~2 neq cm^{-2} h^{-1} (i.e., about 1/1000th the net fluxes of Na^+ or Cl^-) across dog tracheal epithelium that is approximately doubled by epinephrine. Under open-circuit conditions, the baseline net secretion increases to ~4.5 neq cm^{-2} h^{-1}. Surprisingly, submucosal ouabain failed to inhibit Ca^{2+} secretion [434].

2.8.17 Na$^+$-glucose Cotransport

In horse tracheal epithelium, electrogenic Na$^+$-glucose cotransport accounts for ~25% of I$_{sc}$ [435]. This process is absent, however, from primary cultures of human tracheal epithelium [436]. Nevertheless, uptake of glucose across the apical membrane of the latter serves to maintain the glucose concentration of ASL below that of plasma, and is important in preventing bacterial colonization of the airways [436].

2.9   WATER TRANSPORT

Absorption or secretion of water by epithelia is driven by osmotic gradients set up within the epithelium by active solute transport, and these flows of water are believed to take a predominantly transcellular route across even the leakiest of epithelia [437]. In epithelia with the highest rates of isoosmolar fluid absorption (e.g., proximal tubule and salivary gland acini), aquaporins (AQP) mediate most of this transcellular fluid flow [438]. In large human airways, AQP5 is found in the apical membrane and AQP3 in the basolateral [439]. In small human airways, AQP3 is the only AQP present, in the apical membrane [439]. By contrast, in rats and mice, AQP3 and AQP4 are found in the basolateral membrane [440]. Double knock-out of both AQP3 and AQP4 in mice reduced the osmotic permeability of airway epithelium by ~40% [440]. However, neither the depth nor the [Na$^+$] of ASL were altered. Nor was the ability of airway epithelium to hydrate inspired gases [440]. Knock-out of AQP3 alone reduced osmotic permeability to the same extent as double knock-out of AQP3/AQP4. However, removal of fluid instilled into a segment of trachea was unaltered by knock-out of AQP3 [440]. Thus, though present in airway epithelium, AQPs appear to play no significant role in airway fluid balance.

Net volume flows (J_v) have been measured across sheets of tracheal wall, where they are the sum of gland secretion and flows across the surface epithelium. However, under baseline conditions in vitro gland secretion is essentially zero [441], and the net transepithelial volume flows may be taken as being mediated by surface epithelium. In addition, a number of studies have measured volume flows across cultures of surface epithelium.

Several methods have been employed. First, assuming isosmolarity of the transported fluid, volume flows can be estimated from the net open circuit fluxes of Na$^+$ and Cl$^-$ across airway wall. As shown in Table 4 fetal tracheas secrete NaCl at ~0.7 µEq cm^{-2} h^{-1}, which assuming [Na$^+$] of 140 mEq/l and [Cl$^-$] of 120 mEq/l corresponds to ~5 µl cm^{-2} h^{-1}. Adult tracheas absorb Na$^+$ at ~1.5 µEq cm^{-2} h^{-1} and Cl$^-$ at 0.7 µEq cm^{-2} h^{-1}. The reason for the discrepancy between Na$^+$ and Cl$^-$ fluxes is unknown; perhaps a substantial amount of HCO$_3^-$ accompanies the absorbed Na$^+$. The Na$^+$ absorption, if isoosmolar, predicts fluid absorption of ~10 µl cm^{-2} h^{-1}. One study, on dog tracheal epithelium, failed to detect net fluxes of Cl$^-$ and Na$^+$ under open-circuit conditions [324]. However, the dog trachea is unusual in that it shows approximately equal amounts of active

TABLE 4: Net fluxes of Na^+ and Cl^- across open-circuited airway epithelia.

SPECIES	TISSUE	NET J_{Na} (μEq $cm^{-2} h^{-1}$	NET J_{Cl} (μEq $cm^{-2} h^{-1}$)	REF
Pig	Nose (inferior horn)	3.6	—	[309]
Pig	Nose (lower septum)	1.7	—	[309]
Rabbit	Nose	1.2	0.2	[309]
Human	Nose	2.1	—	[309]
Rabbit	Trachea	1.7	0.0	[309]
Rabbit	Trachea	1.7	1.6	[322]
Dog	Trachea	1.0	−0.1	[317]
Dog	Trachea	0.1	−0.3	[324]
Fetal dog	Trachea	−0.7	−0.8	[442]
Sheep	Trachea	1.2	0.8	[315]
Fetal sheep	Trachea	−0.4	−0.7	[315]
Dog	Main-stem Bronchus	0.7	0.1	[317]
Dog	Bronchus (Gen. 4–6)	1.7	1.6	[317]
Sheep	Bronchus	1.4	0.9	[315]
Human	Bronchus	1.2	0.5	[33]

Positive values indicate absorption; negative, secretion.

Cl^- secretion and active Na^+ absorption under baseline conditions [324]; absorption of Na^+ is the predominant active ion transport process in the other adult tissues listed in Table 4.

Several volumetric and gravimetric approaches have been taken to measuring volume flows across airway epithelia. For instance, dog tracheal epithelial cells were grown on the inner surface of a porous "biofiber." One end was plugged, and the lumen filled with saline. Fluid absorption was then estimated from the movement of a meniscus along a constant-bore glass tube attached to the open end. Tracheal cells absorbed liquid at 0.7 $\mu l\ cm^{-2}\ h^{-1}$; bronchial cells, at 2.2 $\mu l\ cm^{-2}\ h^{-1}$ [443]. The same method has been applied to "xenograph" cultures. These are obtained by first removing epithelial cells from rat tracheas. Airway epithelial cells are then seeded into these "denuded" tracheas. Following transplantation under the skin of immune-deficient mouse, seeded human cells formed an intact epithelium that absorbed liquid at ~3 $\mu l\ cm^{-2}\ h^{-1}$ [444]. Pig bronchi filled with physiological saline absorbed liquid at ~4 $\mu l\ cm^{-2}\ h^{-1}$, as determined gravimetrically. Adding Cl^- channel blockers to the luminal liquid had no effect on this fluid absorption suggesting that Cl^- secretion by either surface epithelium or glands was not contributing to net liquid flows [445]. In other studies, 100 μl of saline was added to the mucosal surface of primary cultures of human tracheal epithelium of 5 cm^2 area, and this was then covered with paraffin oil to prevent evaporation [446]. Twenty-four hours later, ~80 μl of saline remained. This corresponds to a rate of fluid absorption of ~0.2 $\mu l\ cm^{-2}\ h^{-1}$. This is markedly lower than obtained with most other techniques. One reason may be that about half the O_2 that airway cells consume enters across the apical membrane [447]. Therefore, though O_2 solubility in paraffin oil is higher than that in water [448], by increasing the length of the diffusion pathway, the paraffin oil may have significantly impaired O_2 supply to the cells.

Another approach involved plugging one end of an isolated segment of pig trachea and suspending it in physiological saline, with the open end above the surface. The lumen was then filled with saline containing dextran blue. From the rate at which the concentration of dextran blue increased, it was calculated that liquid was absorbed at ~35 $\mu l\ cm^{-2}\ h^{-1}$. Absorption was abolished by amiloride, but unaffected by Cl transport inhibitors [449]. It is unclear why this method produces such high estimates of volume absorption. In primary cultures of human tracheal epithelium, measurements of dextran blue concentration in the mucosal liquid yielded rates of volume absorption of ~0.7 $\mu l.\ cm^{-2}\ h^{-1}$ [130].

Airway epithelia have been cultured in the form of fluid-filled spheroids that are bounded by a single cell layer with the ciliated apical cell membrane facing the outside [132]. The rate of increase in volume of the spheroids corresponded to fluid absorption of 3.5 $\mu l\ cm^{-2}\ h^{-1}$. Again, this was completely inhibited by amiloride [132]. In a related approach, fetal rat tracheas were embedded in a collagen gel, in which they sealed up to form roughly spherical structures with the apical membrane facing inwards. From their increases in volume and surface area over an interval of one week a secretion of 1.9 $\mu l\ cm^{-2}\ h^{-1}$ was calculated [450].

We have measured the depth of ASL in sheets of native bovine trachea by low-temperature scanning electron microscopy of tissues rapidly frozen by immersion in liquid N_2 [31]. A 2-min exposure to methacholine increased the depth from 23 to 78 μm. Depth then decreased to 32 μm at 30 min. The initial increase in depth was blocked by bumetanide, an inhibitor of active chloride secretion; we attribute it to gland secretion. The decline in depth between 2 and 30 min was blocked by amiloride, and corresponds to absorption of 9.9 μl cm^{-2} h^{-1}.

Several studies [32, 135, 340] have measured volume flows across airway epithelium or its primary cultures with the dual capacitance probe apparatus first described by Wiedner et al. [451]. In this technique, a sheet of epithelium is mounted between half-chambers that are filled with medium until meniscuses appear within vertical tubes that open into the tops of the half-chambers. A capacitance probe is then placed over each meniscus and is used to detect the distance between the probe tip and the meniscus. As fluid is transported across the epithelium the two probes sense reciprocal changes in capacitance. Each half-chamber has a port that can be used to remove and replace medium. V_{te} is determined with Ag/AgCl electrodes placed close to either side of the cell sheet. Current-passing electrodes at the backs of the chambers can be used to determine R_{te} from deflections in V_{te}. This technique has many advantages: sensitivity in the nanoliter range, excellent time resolution, and simultaneous measurements of V_{te} and R_{te} with J_v.

Using this apparatus, we determined that under baseline conditions, primary cultures of human nasal or tracheal epithelium absorbed fluid at 2.2 and 4.8 μl cm^{-2} h^{-1}, respectively [32]. Amiloride markedly inhibited volume absorption (Figure 24A). In the presence of amiloride, elevation of cAMP (Figure 24A) or [Ca^{2+}]$_i$ (not shown) stimulated fluid secretion to approximately the same degree [32]. However, in the absence of amiloride, the response to elevation of cAMP was frequently an increase in fluid absorption (Figure 24B).

Further studies showed that whether a tissue secreted or absorbed liquid in response to cAMP was determined by V_{te}. In the amiloride-treated tissue illustrated in Figure 24A, V_{te} was −2 mV (lumen negative). In the tissue that did not receive amiloride (Figure 24B), V_{te} was −45 mV. On average, in the absence of amiloride, human tracheal cultures had mean V_{te} of −37 mV, and showed no change in mean volume flow on addition of forskolin (though this agent dramatically reduced V_{te} and R_{te}). Bovine tracheal cultures, by contrast, had markedly higher V_{te} (mean of −67 mV), and in them cAMP elevation increase liquid absorption from 6.0 ± 3.3 to 15.0 ± 3.4 μl cm^{-2} h^{-1} [340]. Furthermore, there was a significant correlation between baseline V_{te} and the cAMP-induced increase in fluid absorption that predicted zero response at −35 mV [340].

The mechanism by which elevation of cAMP increased fluid absorption was investigated further in bovine tracheal cultures. First, it was found that elevation of cAMP did not alter net absorption of Na$^+$ across short-circuited tissues (thus cAMP-stimulated fluid absorption under open-circuit was not due to an increase in active Na$^+$ absorption). Second, net fluid absorption was inhibited by NPPB, the blocker of CFTR (Figure 24B). Third, microelectrode measurements of V_a, indicated that for all V_{te}s of greater than ~35 mV lumen negative, the electrochemical gradient for Cl$^-$ was directed inwardly across the apical membrane. Finally, a cAMP-activated Cl$^-$ channel, that was not CFTR, was demonstrated in the basolateral membrane. Thus, with an inwardly directed

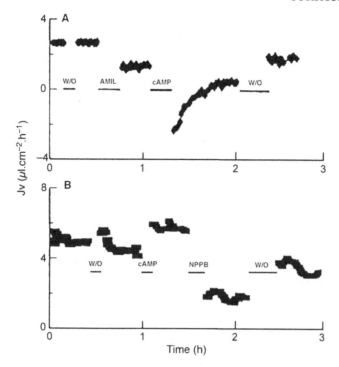

FIGURE 24: Elevation of cAMP can stimulate either secretion or absorption of liquid across primary cultures of human tracheal epithelium. A) A cell sheet was absorbing liquid at ~3 μl cm^{-2} h^{-1}. Changing the medium (w/o) had no effect on J_v. Adding amiloride (AMIL) inhibited J_v. Elevating cAMP with a combination of CPT-cAMP and IBMX induced fluid secretion. Washing out the drugs (w/o) returned J_v towards baseline. B) Baseline absorption was ~5 μl cm^{-2} h^{-1}. Changing the medium (w/o) had little effect. Increasing cAMP with forskolin stimulated absorption, which was inhibited by NPPB (a blocker of CFTR). Washing out the drugs (w/o) then returned J_v towards baseline. Horizontal bars indicate periods when capacitance probes were removed to allow solution changes. Taken from refs. [32, 340].

electrochemical gradient for Cl$^-$ across the apical membrane, cAMP-mediated opening of CFTR causes net entry of Cl$^-$, which exits down a favorable electrochemical gradient through cAMP-activated Cl$^-$ channels in the basolateral membrane [340]. Alternatively, basolateral Cl channels may be activated by the swelling associated with increased influx of Cl$^-$ through CFTR [396]. In either case, the end result is the creation of a route for transepithelial absorption of Cl$^-$ (much as in the sweat duct) and net absorption of NaCl and water is potentiated.

Several general conclusions can be drawn from these measurements of transepithelial volume flows. 1) Fetal airway epithelium secretes fluid under baseline conditions at ~5 μl cm^{-2} h^{-1}. 2) Under baseline conditions, most methods indicate that *adult* airway epithelium absorbs liquid at

~5 μl cm^{-2} h^{-1}, a process driven by amiloride-sensitive active transport of Na$^+$. 3) The effect of opening apical membrane Cl channels (either CFTR or CaCC) depends on V_{te}. At V_{te} of ~−35 mV, there is no change in fluid absorption. At V_{te} less negative than −35 mV, fluid movement shifts in a secretory direction. With V_{te} more negative than ~35 mV, fluid absorption is increased. Thus, Cl$^-$ is actively secreted at V_{te} less negative than 35 mV, and passively absorbed by a transcellular route at more negative V_{te}s.

All these studies were performed with a comparatively large volume of fluid on the mucosal surfaces of the cells. With the capacitance probe technique there were several milliliters of mucosal medium per cm^2 of epithelial surface. In the studies showing amiloride-sensitive reduction of ASL depth following stimulation of gland secretion [31], the mucosal volume was 8 μl cm^{-2}. In biofibers there are ~20 μl cm^{-2} [443], and a similar volume was present in the gravimetric determinations of volume removal from the surface of planar sheets of cultured tracheal epithelium [452]. In vivo, however, the volume of ASL is only ~1 μl cm^{-2}, and it has been argued that changes in the concentration of autocrine agents in this low volume of ASL precisely regulate its depth. This hypothesis will be discussed further in the next section.

2.10   REGULATION OF ASL DEPTH AND SALT CONTENT

Two hypotheses have been advanced as to what determines the depth of ASL (gel and sol combined). As reviewed in the preceding section, measurements of transepithelial volume flows in vitro have invariably shown that adult airway epithelium is absorptive. It was proposed, therefore, that liquid would be absorbed from the airway lumen until some minimal volume was reached at which the remaining liquid was retained in the lumen by forces of surface tension generated by the closely packed cilia and microvilli and by the mucous gel [453]. This hypothesis predicts that with the ASL held in place by forces of surface tension, the continued absorption of salt would generate a [NaCl] in the ASL less than that of plasma [454]. The tendency for water to move down the osmotic pressure gradient from lumen to interstitium would be exactly offset by the forces of surface tension holding it in the lumen. The equilibrium value for [NaCl]$_{ASL}$ would then reflect the balance between the rate at which salt was pumped out and the rate at which NaCl leaked back down its concentration gradient from the interstitium to lumen.

An alternative hypothesis is that, at physiological values of ASL depth, fluid absorption driven by active absorption of Na$^+$ is exactly balanced by fluid secretion driven by active secretion of Cl$^-$ and HCO$_3^-$. Further, this balance is achieved because the concentrations of several agents that modulate transepithelial ion transport are dependent on ASL depth. Specifically, as active Na$^+$ absorption pumps down ASL depth, increases in the concentration of ATP and UTP would inhibit active Na$^+$ absorption [418] while stimulating CaCC-mediated Cl$^-$ secretion. An increase in the concentration of adenosine (produced from the breakdown of ATP) would also stimulate CFTR-dependent Cl^- secretion [455] A number of other factors would inhibit Na^+ absorption including decreased expression of prostatin [234] and increases in the concentration of endogenous protease inhibitors [376] and SPLUNC1 (see Figure 21). Thus, any increase in ASL depth, due say to gland secretion or inflammatory extravasation, would be followed by a decrease in depth driven by active Na^+ absorption across the surface epithelium. However, as depth decreases, Na^+ absorption is turned off and Cl^- secretion is turned on until a precise balance between the fluid flows driven by the two is achieved at the resting depth of ASL of ~10 μm.

One hypothesis predicts that [NaCl] of ASL will be less than that of plasma. The second predicts that it will be the same. So two questions arise. First, what is the [NaCl] of ASL? Second, if liquid were held in place by surface tension, how much lower would the [NaCl] of ASL be than that of plasma?

Dealing with the second question first, if water were held in the lumen by surface tension while NaCl was continuously removed, a rough estimate of the equilibrium value for $[NaCl]_{ASL}$ can be obtained as follows. At equilibrium, the rate at which NaCl is actively removed will equal the rate at which it diffuses back into the lumen down its concentration gradient between interstitium and blood. Fluid absorption of 5 μl cm^{-2} h^{-1} (see Section 2.9) corresponds to active transfer of NaCl/ $NaHCO_3$ of ~0.75 mmol cm^{-2} h^{-1}. The transepithelial concentration gradient at which passive backflux from interstitium to lumen equals active removal in the opposite direction can be estimated from backflux = $P_{NaCl} \cdot \Delta C$, where ΔC is the transepithelial concentration gradient for NaCl. For human bronchial epithelium of ~100 Ω cm^2, under short-circuit conditions the fluxes of Na^+ and Cl^- in the directions opposite to their active transport are ~4 μEq cm^{-2} h^{-1} [33]. Knowing the $[Na^+]$ and $[Cl^-]$ of the physiological saline used, these fluxes can be converted into permeability coefficients. Setting backflux equal to active removal (i.e., 0.75 mmol cm^{-2} h^{-1}), and plugging the estimated values for either P_{Na} or P_{Cl} (the lower of the two should be used, but they are approximately equal) into the equation for backflux predicts a transepithelial NaCl concentration gradient of ~25 mM. In other words, if water were held in the lumen by surface tension, and NaCl were being actively removed, at equilibrium the [NaCl] of ASL would be ~25 mM less than that of plasma. The value of 25 mM was calculated from fluxes measured on tissues with R_{te} of 100 Ω cm^2. This is on the low side for airway epithelia, and for higher resistances the predicted [NaCl] of ASL would be less.

So, what is the [NaCl] of ASL? Multiple studies have used small pieces ("pledgets") of filter paper applied to the luminal surface to collect ASL [456]. What is not often stated in is that the filter paper used is generally about 200 μm thick. Clearly, if applied dry, it will collect fluid from sources other than the underlying ASL [457, 458]. In one study, 5.4 μl of fluid was collected [457], though the volume of ASL under the filter paper (2 × 10 mm) should have been only 0.2 μl (assuming a depth of 10 μm). It is possible that much of the extra fluid was ASL from regions adjacent to the filter paper. However, plasma markers were detected in the collected fluid, and it was concluded that "absorbing discs severely disturb the epithelial-barrier function and sample subepithelial fluid and solutes" [457]. The discs may also damage the cells themselves; the $[K^+]$ in filter paper samples is often considerably higher than $[K^+]$ predicted for passive distribution according to V_{te}. Even if the epithelial cells were not structurally damaged, the mechanical irritation could induce secretion of Cl^- and water.

One approach to circumventing these problems is to use filter paper pieces pre-equilibrated with physiological saline and allow sufficient time (~2 h) for them to equilibrate with the ASL [427]. A second is to use ashless filter paper, which takes up smaller volumes of liquid [459]. Pledgets of this kind of paper, 4 cm in length and 5 mm in width, took up an average of 20 μl of fluid from the surface of people's noses. However, the catalogue states that the filter paper used is 200 μm thick. The total volume of a pledget is therefore 4000 μl! In the most recent reincarnation of this general approach, lens paper was fused to Parafilm. This has the advantage that there will be no evaporation from the surface distant from the ASL. The thickness of the paper was not specified, but 3 μl of liquid per cm^2 of surface was collected, a value not markedly greater than the expected volume of ASL under the paper. Values of $[NaCl]_{ASL}$ determined with filter paper are usually close to those of plasma [286, 459]. However, when sampled with filter paper pre-equilibrated with saline, the $[Na^+]$ of equine tracheal ASL (127 mEq/l) was significantly less than plasma, while the $[K^+]$ (17 mEq/l) was significantly higher [427].

Collection of ASL with microcapillaries [456] shares many of the problems associated with the use of filter paper [458]. Investigators have also used "miniature" Na-selective glass electrodes [459] to measure $[Na^+]_{ASL}$. But these have a tip diameter of 1.2 mm, which is quite large compared to the depth of the ASL on which the measurements are being made. Cl-sensing Ag/AgCl wires of 127 μm diameter have also been used [460]. They are encased in polyethylene tubing with a 2-mm length of naked wire protruding. As for filter paper, all these various probes detect $[Na^+]$ and $[Cl^-]$ in ASL similar to those of plasma, but again the possibility of damage to the epithelium cannot be entirely excluded.

Ion-sensitive microelectrodes are perhaps the least invasive and most accurate means of determining ASL ion contents. They also have the advantage that ASL ion concentrations can be monitored continuously, and any changes in response to pharmacological manipulation of ion transport determined. However, they only seem to have been used twice on ASL. In one study, primary cultures of human airway epithelium were used that were grown on 4.5 cm^2 inserts and had $R_{te} >$ 300 Ω cm^2. After washing three times with PBS, 200 μl of PBS added to the apical surface. Thirty-six or 48 h later, Cl^--selective microelectrodes showed $[Cl]_{ASL}$ not significantly different from that of the bathing media [461]. Given that fluid absorption across airway epithelium is ~5 μl cm^{-2} h^{-1} (see above), the ASL should have recovered from the earlier addition of PBS, but it is puzzling that

TABLE 5: Estimates of [Na$^+$] and [Cl$^-$] of ASL made with fluorescence microscopy.

TISSUE	[Na]$_{ASL}$ (mEq/l)	[Cl]$_{ASL}$ (mEq/l)	REF
Bovine tracheal epithelial culture	97	118	[341]
Mouse trachea	115	140	[341]
Human bronchi	103	92	[341]
Mouse distal airway	122	123	[463]

no measurements were reported for tissues that had been undisturbed by addition of PBS. A second study, with ion-selective microelectrodes, showed that [K$^+$] of ASL was ~20 mEq/l [427].

In a radioisotopic approach to determining the ion contents of ASL, ^{36}Cl and ^{3}H$_2$O (or ^{22}Na and ^{3}H$_2$O) were added to the basolateral side of primary cultures of human airway epithelium, and allowed to pass across the epithelium and equilibrate with the ASL [462]. The ASL was collected by flushing the mucosal surface with PBS, and [Cl$^-$] and [Na$^+$] calculated from the ratio of ^{36}Cl to ^{3}H$_2$O or ^{22}Na to ^{3}H$_2$O, respectively. [Na$^+$] and [Cl$^-$] concentrations of ASL were determined to be 50 and 40 mEq/l, respectively. It is notable that the tissues had comparatively high values for both active Na$^+$ absorption and R_{te}; exactly the conditions favoring reduction of [NaCl]$_{ASL}$. However, the high water permeability of airway epithelium makes this radioisotopic approach difficult to perform. Though the medium used to obtain the ASL was purportedly present for exactly 3 sec between addition and removal, the permeability of the epithelium to water is so high that even a difference of a second or two makes an appreciable difference in the amount of ^{3}H$_2$O collected. These experiments should be repeated with a less permeant marker of the extracellular space such as [^{3}H]-mannitol.

Microscopical approaches have recently been used to determine the ion contents of ASL. In brief, fluorescent probes for Na$^+$, Cl$^-$ or K$^+$ are added to ASL in the least invasive manner possible, either as a powder or as a small aliquot of concentrated stock solution. The tissue is allowed to recover, and ion concentrations are then determined by fluorescence microscopy. The results are summarized in Table 5. Given that [K$^+$] of ASL is ~20 mEq/l [381], and there will be some HCO$_3^-$ present, these values are consistent with ASL being approximately isoosmolar with plasma.

Measurements of airway surface liquid osmolarity by fluorescence microscopy confirm this prediction. Liposomes containing calcein, a self-quenching fluorophore that responds to changes in liposome volume were added to ASL, with the volume of liposome suspension (46 nl/cm^2) being small compared the volume of ASL (2.2 μl/cm^2). The osmolarity of ASL over primary cultures of bovine tracheal epithelium was estimated as 325 ± 12 mOsm. In mouse trachea, it was 330 ± 36 mOsm [464].

Thus, the balance of the evidence strongly suggests that ASL has essentially the same composition as plasma. Does, then, the equilibrium depth of ASL reflect a balance between active Na$^+$ absorption and active Cl$^-$ secretion?

Several studies have described the effects of pharmacologically manipulating active Na$^+$ absorption or active Cl$^-$ secretion on the depth of ASL as determined by confocal fluorescence microscopy. Inhibition of Cl$^-$ secretion with bumetanide reduces the depth over cultures of human tracheal epithelium from 7.5 to ~3 μm [465], and a combination of blockers of CFTR or CaCC reduces ASL depth by about the same amount [466]. Stimulation of cAMP-dependent Cl$^-$ secretion with adenosine or forskolin increases ASL depth by 50–100% [465, 467], with the effects of forskolin being blocked by an inhibitor of CFTR [467]. Interestingly, amiloride only increases ASL depth from 8 to 10 μm [467]. This suggests that there is little active Cl$^-$ secretion under baseline conditions, and is therefore inconsistent with the effects of bumetanide. Similar results have been obtained with pieces of tracheal wall from both pigs and humans. Amiloride or elevation of cAMP both approximately doubled the depth of ASL, and the effects of cAMP elevation were blocked by an inhibitor of CFTR [467].

The extent to which the in vitro results are applicable in vivo is questionable, however. In the primary cultures used in the measurements of ASL V_{te} has generally been ~−10 mV [465]. This is considerably less than the value of ~−30 mV measured in vivo for human trachea [303, 305, 308]. Lower V_{te}s favor Cl$^-$ secretion, which may therefore be greater in vitro then in vivo. It is true that in some studies in vivo V_{te}s were determined with probes that made contact with the airway surface by emitting a continuous stream of physiological saline [303, 305]. Thus, any autocrine agents regulating ASL depth would have been considerably diluted. However, similar values were independently obtained with a solid exploring electrode [308].

In fact, for tracheas in vivo, with V_{te} of ~30 mV, it seems that there will be little active Cl$^-$ secretion; Cl$^-$ is close to equilibrium across the apical membrane, and Cl$^-$ secretion can only be in-duced transiently by elevation of either cAMP or [Ca^{2+}]$_i$ (see Section 2.8.4). However, the very presence of the V_{te} indicates that there are substantial amounts of active Na$^+$ absorption. Smaller airways have smaller V_{te}s, and possibly, therefore, more Cl$^-$ secretion under open-circuit conditions. However, nothing is known about their membrane potentials.

Though active Na$^+$ absorption and active Cl$^-$ secretion undoubtedly affect ASL depth, forces of surface tension may ultimately prevent complete removal of liquid no matter what ion transport processes are operating. Thus, nystatin induces continuous high levels of Na^+ absorption that are presumably not affected by changes in concentration of ASL components. Nystatin would therefore be expected to result in complete absorption of ASL. However, instead it reduces ASL depth from 8 to 4 μm [468]. Under no circumstances yet reported has ASL been removed completely.

Much of the evidence that ASL depth is determined by the balance between active Na^+ absorption and active Cl^- secretion comes from work with CF cell cultures. These obviously lack cAMP-dependent Cl^- secretion, and it has been reported that active absorption of Na^+ is elevated [314], and, as expected, it was found that ASL depth was less than normal in CF airway cell cultures [461, 466]. This finding, however, has not been confirmed by more recent investigations from other groups [469, 470]. These studies are discussed in more detail in Section 4.4.5.

Primary cultures of CF airway epithelium show a complete failure of mucociliary transport [461, 471]. However, children with CF have detectable rates of mucociliary clearance [472]. The shear stresses imparted on airway epithelium in vivo by tidal volume expansion and airflow may account for this discrepancy. Thus, when cyclical shear stresses were applied to primary cultures of human tracheal epithelium the depth of ASL over CF cultures was increased and mucociliary clearance rates similar to those of non-CF cells were induced [466]. Shear stress induced release of ATP across the cells' apical membranes, and it was proposed that the resulting inhibition of Na^+ absorption coupled with a stimulation of Ca-dependent Cl^- secretion accounted for the increase in ASL depth. Shear stress also increased ASL depth over non-CF cultures [455].

A number of points may be made to summarize this section. First, there is no doubt that Cl^- secretion across airway epithelium promotes an increase in ASL depth, whereas active Na^+ absorption promotes a decrease. Second, however, the studies with nystatin indicate that forces of surface tension do play a role in retaining fluid in the airway lumen. The greater the level of Na^+ absorption relative to Cl^- secretion, the less may be the ASL depth. But even when levels of Na^+ absorption are artificially high and incapable of being regulated, ASL is not completely removed. Third, the measurements of $[Na^+]$ in ASL determined with fluorescence microscopy show it be 20 to 40 mEq/L less than plasma (Table 5). This is consistent with the pumping of Na^+ out of ASL that is held in place by surface tension. Yet, fourth, the osmolarity of ASL is the same as plasma within experimental error. This is because, fifth, the negative V_{te}, coupled with active secretion, results in an increase in the $[K^+]$ of ASL (relative to plasma) that is approximately equal the decrease in its $[Na^+]$ [381, 427]. Finally, the negative V_{te} resulting primarily from active Na^+ absorption would be expected to drive Cl^- out of the lumen by passive diffusion via the paracellular pathway. However, any drop in the $[Cl^-]$ of ASL will shift the electrochemical driving force for Cl^- across the apical membrane in an outward direction, and induce or enhance active transepithelial Cl^- secretion. The $[Cl^-]$ of ASL therefore reflects a balance between the active and passive transport pathways for this anion.

2.11   MUCOCILIARY CLEARANCE

The ciliary beat cycle is illustrated in Figure 25. In their active (propulsive) stroke, cilia beat toward the mouth, and in the middle of this stroke, they stick straight up from the airway surface. Shortly before this point, it is believed that the small claws in the tips of the cilia engage with the underside of the mucus blanket and drag it orally. At the end of the effective stroke the cilia lie flat on the airway surface. There is now a variable pause, the "rest phase." The cilia then enter the "recovery stroke" during which they move backward and to the right parallel and close to the airway surface until they return to the starting point of the effective stroke. In moving backward during their recovery stroke the shafts of the cilia hit the tips of resting cilia, stimulating then to begin their own recovery strokes. Thus, a "metachronal" wave of ciliary activity passes backwards at an obtuse angle (135 degrees) to the right of the effective stroke [3].

Airway cilia beat at 10–20 Hz [1]. The recovery stroke and the rest phase are approximately equal in duration, but the effective stroke is much shorter [473]. Changes in ciliary beat frequency (CBF) generally involve approximately equal changes in the durations of the rest phase and the recovery stroke; the active stroke is comparatively little affected. For instance, when, in cultures of rabbit tracheal epithelium, CBF was increased from ~10 to ~30 Hz by manipulating $[Ca^{2+}]_i$, the decreases in the duration of recovery stroke, rest phase and active stroke were 71%, 77% and 37%, respectively [473]. A large number of neurohumoral mediators increase CBF by elevating either

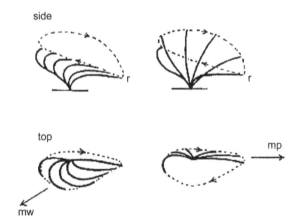

FIGURE 25: The ciliary beat cycle. Seen from the side (top panels) or the top (bottom panels). In the recovery stroke (left panels), the cilium starts from the rest position (r) and moves backward in a clockwise direction. In the effective stroke (right panels), the cilium moves in a plane perpendicular to the airway surface, becoming maximally extended at midstroke. The metachronal wave of beating activity (mw) passes at an angle of ~135° to the direction of the active stroke and mucus propulsion (mp). Taken from ref. [3].

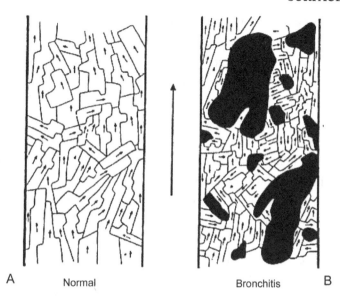

FIGURE 26: Ciliary beat fields in the rat trachea. A) In health. B) Following the induction of mucous metaplasia. Arrows indicate direction of the propulsive stroke in each field. Black areas indicate fields in which cilia are not beating. The large arrow in the center of the figure points cephelad. Taken from ref. [480].

intracellular Ca^{2+} or cAMP [1, 474]. The effects described for cell cultures or isolated cells are quite small with increases in frequency being generally ~25%, and rarely more than 50% [1]. By contrast, a number of the same agents tested on dogs or baboons in vivo show increases in CBF between 100% and 200% [1]. Possibly, in vivo, gland secretions stimulate CBF by altering the rheology of the mucous blanket. The only neurohumoral agonist reported to decrease CBF is adenosine [475]. This agent raises intracellular cAMP levels, but the same group found that a permeable analogue of cAMP stimulated CBF [476].

In cultures of rabbit tracheal epithelium deformation of the apical membrane of a single cell raised its $[Ca^{2+}]_i$ and increased its CBF by ~75%. Then, after a delay of around 0.5 sec, CBF increased in neighboring cells. A wave of increased $[Ca^{2+}]_i$ and ciliary beating eventually spread for long distances over the epithelium [477]. These waves are generated by passage of IP_3 between cells via gap junctions [478].

As shown in Figure 26A, cilia beat in coordinated fields of between a handful and several hundred cells [479]. The exact direction of the propulsive stroke varies from field to field, though in all fields it is directed more cranially than caudally. In experimentally induced mucous metaplasia, the fields become smaller, some start to beat caudally, and some cease beating altogether (Figure 26B).

Mucus transport rates vary with the techniques used to determine them, but in central airways, the least invasive techniques yield values of ~4 mm/min [1]. Interestingly, in rats, the mucous transport rate declines progressively by approximately ten-fold in moving from the trachea to terminal bronchioles [480]. Two factors contribute to this decline. First, the cilia in the distal airways are shorter than in the trachea (~4 μm vs. 7 μm), and their "beat amplitude" (the distance travelled by the tip of a cilium during its active stroke) is ~1.2 μm as opposed to ~10 μm in the trachea [480]. Second, beat frequencies in terminal bronchioles are only ~40% those in the central airways [481]. Functionally, the increase in mucous transport rate up the airways helps prevent flooding with mucous secretions travelling up from lower in the lungs [482].

The rate at which mucus is transported depends on its viscosity and a number of other rheological properties such as elasticity, rigidity, surface tension and spinnability [483, 484]. However, the main determinant of all these parameters may be the degree of hydration (i.e., the mucus concentration) [485]. Too much or too little water in the mucus gel can markedly reduce mucus transport velocities. This is dramatically illustrated by studies on pig bronchi in which acetylcholine increased mucociliary transport three-fold. A variety of experiments showed that this was due to gland secretion rather than goblet cell discharge or increased CBF [486, 487]. However, if gland liquid secretion was inhibited with Cl^- channel blockers, then in response to acetylcholine glands produced an abnormally condensed and viscous mucous blanket that resulted in slowing rather than acceleration of mucociliary transport [486–488]. This slowing could, however, be partly mitigated by inhibiting liquid absorption across the surface epithelium [486].

At birth, the mucous blanket is presumably absent, and the same may be true of healthy adults breathing exceptionally clean air. A report of airway mucus being present in the form of isolated rafts [489] could therefore be regarded as representing a stage in the development of a complete mucous blanket. In a recent study, however, it has been proposed that such rafts may form from a continuous blanket during normal mucociliary clearance [490]. Thus, it was found that when particles fall on a thin mucus gel, the mucus collapses round them. Next the mucus sticks to the cilia, and their beating bundles the gel into discrete strands of mucus. This somehow stimulates further mucus secretion and a complete (and less sticky) mucus gel is generated. It was suggested that increased sticking of mucus to cilia could contribute to mucus accumulation in airway disease.

CHAPTER 3

Airway Glands

The structure and function of airway glands have been reviewed [136, 441, 491, 492]. No more than a brief synopsis is provided here.

All tracheobronchial glands secrete mucus. They are "tubuloacinar," a structure akin to a bunch of grapes, in which acini are connected to tubules, which then fuse several times before emptying into a single large "terminal duct" that is about 1 mm long in adults and opens to the airway surface [29, 493, 494]. There are about 100 acini in most adult human tracheal glands. The exact form of the glands depends on where they lie in relation to the cartilaginous rings (i.e., on how much space they have in which to grow). Directly over the middle of rings, glands are shaped like pancakes. Between the rings, they are elongate and symmetrical. Growing over the sloping side of a ring, they become markedly asymmetrical (Figure 27).

In the adult human trachea and main bronchi, gland openings occur at ~1 per mm^2 of airway surface, and the aggregate gland volume is ~15 μl per cm^2 of airway surface [21, 28]. Thus, individual glands have an average volume of ~150 nl. However, both the frequency and size of glands declines with increasing airway generation until they disappear at ~generation 8 [21], at which point the airway internal diameter is ~2 mm. Glands also disappear at airways of about this size in pig and sheep [495, 496].

In most of the larger mammals studied (ox, pig, sheep, dog, goat), frequency, aggregate volume and individual size of tracheal glands are similar to those of the human trachea [28]. In the horse trachea, however, glands are comparatively much smaller and fewer than in other large mammals [57] presumably because, as mentioned earlier, this species is an obligate nose breather with large and complex nasal turbinates. In mammals of intermediate size (e.g., cat, ferret, rhesus monkey), the tracheal gland density remains ~1 per mm^2, but the size of the individual glands is less than that in humans [28]. In the rat and the guinea pig, glands are present throughout the trachea but at reduced frequency and lower volume [26]. The rabbit trachea, however, lacks glands [26], perhaps for the same reasons as suggested above for the horse. Finally, in the smallest mammals, tracheal glands, if present, are very small and found in small numbers at the junction with the larynx [26,

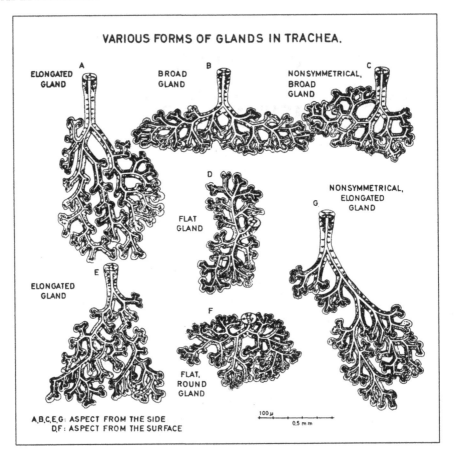

FIGURE 27: Various gland structures in fetal human trachea. Glands in adult trachea are similar in basic structure, but the length of the terminal ducts and the numbers of acini are several fold greater. Taken from ref. [29].

497, 498]. When, for eleven mammalian species (excluding the horse), the overall volume of glands per unit area of tracheal surface was plotted against tracheal diameter, the relationship was linear with glands disappearing at an airway internal diameter of ~1–2 mm [57], the same diameter at which glands disappear in the tracheobronchial tree of humans, pigs and sheep [21, 495, 496].

The nose contains submucosal glands similar to those of the tracheobronchial tree, and their distribution roughly parallels the pattern of particle distribution [499]. However, they are found at almost ten times the frequency of tracheobronchial glands [500, 501], and are only about one quarter the size [502]. Similar small glands are found at low frequency (~0.1 to 0.5 per mm^2) in the nasal sinuses [503]. In addition, the nose contains a number of specialized glands. Bowman's glands of the olfactory epithelium do not secrete gel-forming mucins, and are believed to provide liquid to dissolve inhaled odorants [504]. Similar glands are found in the vomeronasal and septal olfactory organs [505]. Though vestigial in humans, in many other vertebrates these glands serve to detect pheromones. Anterior nasal glands consist of scattered groups of acini that open into a duct of several centimeters in length that terminates at the nostrils [504, 506]. They are involved in humidification of inspired air, heat regulation and odorant presentation [507, 508].

Submucosal gland acini are lined with serous cells. These are characterized by small electron-dense granules, generally of 100 to 300 nm in diameter [96, 509]. There is abundant structural and physiological evidence that serous cells secrete liquid [441, 510]. They also secrete a wide range of antimicrobials, anti-inflammatory agents and compounds involved in the innate immune response [441, 511]. Of the antimicrobials, lactoferrin and lysozyme are quantitatively the most important. The secretory tubules are lined with mucous cells [96, 509] that contain electron-lucent granules, which average considerably larger than the opaque granules of serous cells. The granules are densely packed with little cytoplasm between them, and the nucleus is pushed down into the very base of the cell. The major constituent of these granules is MUC5B [169]. Several recent studies indicate that mucous cells may also contribute to gland liquid secretions [441, 512]. Figure 28 illustrates the basic ultrastructural differences between these two cell types.

The acini and secretory tubules are surrounded by a discontinuous sheath of myoepithelial cells [514] that probably provides structural support to counteract the intraluminal hydrostatic pressure that develops during gland liquid secretion.

Secretory tubules may fuse several times before emptying into the distal portion of the terminal duct, a region that is often dilated to form the so-called collecting duct [493]. In pig trachea about ~25% of glands have collecting ducts [494]. The percentage of glands that have collecting ducts in humans is unknown, and it is possible that these structures appear only during high rates of gland secretion. Nevertheless, the epithelial histology of the distal and proximal portions of the terminal duct differs; the proximal portion has a mucociliary histology resembling that of the surface epithelium [96, 509, 515], and is often referred to as the "ciliated duct." The distal portion is lined with non-ciliated pseudostratified columnar epithelium, the exact form of which depends on species [96, 509, 515].

In airway glands, volume secretion is driven by a combination of Cl^- and HCO_3^- secretion [291, 516–520]. All evidence indicates that active Cl^- secretion by airway glands is by the same ubiquitous Na^+-linked mechanism common to all vertebrate epithelia, as described earlier for the surface epithelium. However, the predominant Cl^- channel in the apical membrane of gland serous cells is CaCC rather than CFTR [512, 517, 518]. Calcium-activated bicarbonate secretion involves generation of HCO_3^- and H^+ by carbonic anhydrase coupled to efflux of HCO_3^- through CaCC and extrusion of H^+ via a basolateral Na^+/H^+ exchanger [519]. By contrast, in cAMP-dependent

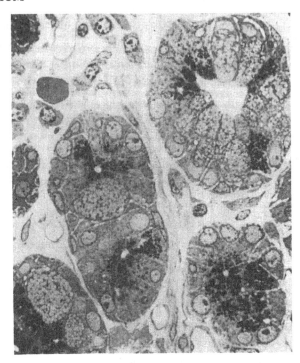

FIGURE 28: Section through ferret tracheal glands showing profiles of several serous acini (small lumens, electron-dense granules) and a mucous tubule (top right; large lumen, electron-lucent granules). Taken from ref. [513].

HCO_3^- secretion, HCO_3^- efflux across the apical membrane is exclusively via CFTR, with some of the HCO_3^- being generated by carbonic anhydrase and some entering the cells on a basolateral DIDS-sensitive Na^+/HCO_3^- cotransporter [519].

Maximal fluid flows from tracheal glands are 10–20 nl/min [30, 521–525]. With one gland per mm^2, this means that the maximal levels of secretion into the airway lumen are 60–120 $\mu l \, cm^{-2} \, h^{-1}$, considerably greater than the rate at which surface epithelium absorbs water (5 $\mu l \, cm^{-2} \, h^{-1}$). Maximal gland secretion can therefore double the depth of ASL within approximately 1 min [31]. The ionic composition of gland secretions is little different from that of plasma [525, 526]. Their pH has been given as either 6.97 [526] or 7.18 [288]. In samples obtained from individual glands, the concentrations of mucin, lactoferrin and lysozyme were 395, 549, and 231 $\mu g/ml$, respectively [206].

Airway glands are innervated primarily by neurons intrinsic to the airway wall, though they also receive input from recurrent axons of C fiber afferents, which release substance P [103]. There are approximately equal numbers of adrenergic and cholinergic nerve terminals in the vicinity of human glands [527, 528]. In the cat, by contrast, within 10 μm of glands, cholinergic varicosities are ten times as frequent as adrenergic [529]. In both human and cats, occasional cholinergic terminals penetrate the basement membrane of the glands, but adrenergic nerves do not [528, 529]. VIP-containing neurons are also found in immediate proximity to human airway glands [530]. At least ten other neurotransmitters have been found in nerve terminals adjacent to glands [531]. As reviewed elsewhere [531, 532], glands have been shown to possess receptors for most of these transmitters.

There is an extensive literature on neurohumoral control of airway gland secretion [1, 136, 441]. Whether gland secretion is measured from volume flows, mucin secretion or output of serous cell macromolecules, the same general conclusions apply. First, vagal stimulation induces much higher levels of gland secretion than does sympathetic nerve stimulation [49, 533]. Similarly, exogenous cholinergic agents are much more potent secretagogues than β-adrenergic agents [30, 534, 535]. In most species, α-adrenergic agents have trivial effects on secretion, but in cats and ferrets they are almost as effective as cholinergic agents [30, 525]. VIP is about half as efficacious as cholinergic agents at stimulating gland secretion [524, 536]. VIP and acetylcholine act through different second messengers (Ca^{2+} and cAMP, respectively), and synergize with one another [524, 537]. The effectiveness of substance P as a gland secretagogue varies greatly between species, and it is not particularly important in humans [523, 538]. In addition to autonomic agonists, a wide variety of neurohumoral and inflammatory mediators, and toxic insults stimulate (or occasionally inhibit) gland secretion. Wanner [1] provides a very complete list of the various secretagogues.

An important concept is that receptors for the various autonomic agonists are differentially distributed between serous and mucous cells, and the composition and properties of gland mucus therefore depends on the particular autonomic stimulus. Beta-adrenergic receptors are more numerous on mucous than serous cells, and α1 receptors are more numerous on serous than mucous cells [539]. In the cat, the relative effectiveness as stimulators of gland fluid secretion is in the order cholinergic ≈ α-adrenergic >> β-adrenergic (30, 525). By contrast, as stimulators of mucin secretion the potency sequence is cholinergic > α-adrenergic > β-adrenergic [49, 540–542]. As predicted from these values, the mucin content [525], protein content [543] and viscosity [544] of secretions sampled from individual tracheal glands all depend on the inducing mediators in the sequence β-adrenergic > cholinergic > α-adrenergic. In short, β-adrenergic agents act predominantly on mucous cells to produce a small volume of highly concentrated gland secretions, whereas α-adrenergic agents act predominantly on serous cells to produce a copious amount of dilute secretion. Cholinergic agonists act more evenly on both cell types to produce large volumes of secretions of intermediate mucus concentration. Interestingly, cholinergically mediated secretions have the same viscosity and mucin concentration as basal secretions [525, 543, 544], suggesting that baseline secretion is due to cholinergic tone.

More recently, it has been argued that it is not the mediator, but the flow rate that determines the concentration of gland secretions [545]. Thus, in pig and human bronchi, VIP or forskolin produced low volumes of concentrated secretions, whereas methacholine produced high volumes of dilute secretions. However, when volume flows were manipulated with transport blockers, and when the percent solids was plotted against flow rate for all experimental conditions, the points for VIP, forskolin and methacholine fell on the same line. In other words, at the same flow rates the different mediators induced secretions with the same percent of solids. However, in the cat, for the same flow rates, α-adrenergic and cholinergic agents produce gland secretions of very different composition and viscosity [525, 543, 544].

CHAPTER 4

Pathology

4.1 SOME GENERAL CONSIDERATIONS

In terms of the airway epithelium, all inflammatory airway diseases share some common features: Goblet cell metaplasia and hyperplasia, squamous metaplasia, depression of ciliary beating, slowing of mucus transport, increased permeability of surface epithelium, plasma transudation, leukocyte transmigration, gland hypertrophy, and plugging of the airways with "mucous" secretions [1, 546–549].

However, there are important differences in, among other things, the relative amounts of squamous and mucous metaplasia, the types of leukocytes migrating into the airway lumen, the degree of breakdown in barrier function, the composition of the mucous plugs, and the presence or absence of bacterial infection. Squamous metaplasia is most prevalent in COPD [550]. The eosinophil is the most frequent leukocyte infiltrating the airways in mild to moderate asthma, though neutrophils become important in severe asthma [547]. In COPD, macrophages and neutrophils both greatly outnumber eosinophils [547]. Cystic fibrosis is characterized by massive influx of neutrophils [551]. Differences in the types or amounts of chemokines released by the epithelium [269, 552] are presumably largely responsible for disease-specific differences in leukocyte infiltration. However, the relative contributions of altered extracellular milieu and intrinsic differences in the epithelium are unclear. In this regard, there has been much speculation that airway epithelium in CF is "hyperinflammatory"; it may generate abnormally high levels of pro-inflammatory mediators both in the presence and absence of inflammatory insults [553]. Of the various airway diseases, asthma may be the one with the greatest breakdown in the epithelial barrier [554], and the peculiar rubbery consistency of the mucous plugs seen in status asthmaticus may be due to high levels of plasma proteins [546]. In asthma and COPD, it is likely that the mucin concentration of mucus secreted by either glands or surface epithelium is normal. By contrast, in cystic fibrosis, lack of Cl^- secretion may lead to abnormally high mucin concentrations in gland secretions [526], a problem that may be exacerbated by increased water absorption across the surface epithelium [32]. By inhibiting endogenous antimicrobials, the acidification of ASL consequent on lack of CFTR-mediated HCO_3^- secretion may also contribute to the rampant microbial infections characteristic of CF [286]. Lack of HCO_3^- may also contribute to pathology by hindering the expansion of mucous granules following their release from goblet or gland mucous cells [555].

Changes in epithelial function in the individual diseases are discussed in more detail in the sections that immediately follow. First, however, a brief discussion on how gland hypertrophy and mucus plugging have been quantified is provided.

The index of gland size of most use to the physiologist is the ratio of gland volume to unit area of airway surface. This is identical to the area of gland profiles per unit length of surface epithelium in a transverse section [21], and can be obtained by point-counting [21] or gravimetric analysis [28] performed on projections of standard histological cross-sections. Recently, this measure of gland volume has become readily obtainable by stereology [556]. Another fairly useful measure is total gland volume [557], which can be obtained in the same ways, but is not normalized to airway surface. Unfortunately, both these measures have been comparatively seldom used.

Instead, most early studies used the "Reid Index" to quantify gland hypertrophy in airway diseases. In this approach, on a projection of a cross-section of airway wall, a line is drawn perpendicularly from the epithelium to the outer surface of a cartilaginous ring. The length of this line that lies over profiles of glands (so-called gland thickness) is divided by the line's total length ("wall thickness") to yield the Reid Index [558]. As a measure of gland volume, the Reid Index has the advantage over gland thickness in that it is not affected if sections are oblique rather than perpendicular [559]. However, the primary advantage of the Reid Index is that it can be obtained more easily and quickly than other more sophisticated estimates of gland hypertrophy. Some disadvantages can be identified [560]. First, both wall and gland thickness vary with distance along any profile of a cartilage, and the choice of where to draw the line is often quite subjective. Second, the Reid Index ignores the glands between the cartilaginous plates. This is where most glands are, and glands here show a relatively greater increase in volume in disease than do glands over the cartilaginous plates (Jang & Widdicombe unpublished). Third, if the thickness of the collagenous tissue increases due to edema, as occurs in asthma [561], then even though glands hypertrophy, the Reid Index may not change (or even potentially decrease).

Can reported values of the Reid Index be converted into physiologically more meaningful measures of gland volume? The answer is yes, but only if glands increase in thickness without change in the thickness of the surrounding connective tissue. This is true of chronic bronchitis, where gland thickness can be calculated from the relationship: Reid Index = Gland thickness / (Gland thickness + 0.3) [559]. However, edema, as occurs in asthma, will reduce the Reid Index obtained for any particular gland thickness. Thus, the Reid Index seriously underestimates the degree of gland hypertrophy expressed as volume per unit area, but it is often hard to say by exactly how much.

A second historical approach to measuring gland volume was to calculate the percentage of wall volume, occupied by glands, "gland %," in a histological section [560]. The dependence of Reid Index on gland % is hyperbolic, so the latter is a more sensitive index of hypertrophy. Further, FEV_1 shows significant negative correlation with gland % but not Reid Index [562]. However, gland %

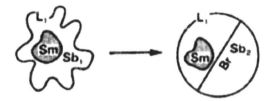

Mucus occupying ratio

Sm/Sb$_2$

FIGURE 29: The mucus occupying ratio (MOR). Left diagram—With a digitizing computer, the area occupied by mucus (Sm), the length of the basement membrane (L$_1$), and the luminal area (Sb$_1$) are estimated. Right diagram—The luminal area (Sb$_2$) and diameter (Br) are then estimated assuming a perfect circle of perimeter, L$_1$. Taken from ref. [563].

shares, with the Reid Index, the disadvantage that it is affected by changes in the dimensions of components of the lung wall other than glands. And, as for the Reid Index, it is impossible to convert into absolute gland volume or volume per unit area.

Though mucous plugging of airways is characteristic of all inflammatory airway diseases, it was not until 1989 that this was put on a quantitative basis when Aikawa et al. [563] defined the mucus occupying ratio (MOR). These authors pointed out that airways collapsed to varying extents on fixation leading, in an airway cross-section, to a drop in the ratio of luminal area to airway perimeter. To correct for this, they measured the perimeter of collapsed airways, and then estimated the area of the airway lumen assuming it to be a circle with the same perimeter. The area of mucus plugs divided by the estimated circular area, or "relaxed area," was termed the "mucus-occupying ratio" (see Figure 29).

4.2 CHRONIC BRONCHITIS

Chronic bronchitis has been defined as: "the condition of subjects with chronic or recurrent excessive mucus secretion in the bronchial tree" [564]. It is one of the two main forms of COPD, a chronic (and usually progressive) increase in the resistance to airflow. The other form of COPD is emphysema. This involves progressive destruction of alveoli, and the loss of their tethering action causes constriction of the small airways. Chronic bronchitis and emphysema usually occur together, and are generally caused by smoking, though other atmospheric pollutants can cause COPD.

In chronic bronchitis, the MOR of "central" airways (i.e., those with cartilage) is increased to ~4% from the normal value of <1%. In "peripheral" airways (i.e., those lacking cartilage) the increase is from <1% in health to ~20% in disease [563]. Thus, chronic bronchitis is predominantly a disease of the small airways.

A peculiar feature of the surface epithelium in COPD is extensive areas of squamous metaplasia in addition to mucous metaplasia. In one particularly thorough study [565], two biopsies were taken from the subsegmental carinae of each of 72 smokers with COPD. The length of intact epithelium in the resulting histological sections averaged 1 mm. Regions of mucous metaplasia were found in all subjects, but squamous metaplasia in only ~45%. However, though mucous metaplasia never accounted for more than 40% of the epithelium, in seven subjects, squamous metaplasia accounted for 50–100% of the epithelium. The impression gained from these numbers is that both mucous and squamous metaplasia are focal. However, the former is found in numerous small foci, the latter in fewer and larger. Squamous metaplasia is seen to a similar degree in both cartilaginous and non-cartilaginous airways [566], and the extent of squamous metaplasia correlates with disease severity [567, 568]. Studies on a cell culture model suggest that squamous metaplasia is associated with increased secretion of IL-1β by the epithelium. This in turn stimulates adjacent fibroblasts to activate TGF-β, and this cytokine induces the production of collagen by fibroblasts resulting in thickening of small airway walls and occlusion of the lumen [568]. Small airway epithelium may contribute to this pathology by itself releasing abnormally high amounts of TGF-β in COPD [569].

In post-mortem specimens of trachea, main and lobar bronchi, goblet cell numbers were increased by ~35% in chronic bronchitis [570]. In bronchoscopy specimens from "large" airways of chronic smokers, the volume of individual goblet cells was increased by 30% and their numbers by 80%, resulting in a 120% increase in the amount of epithelial mucin per unit surface area. Further, the mucus volume was greater in smokers with COPD than those without [571]. Others have confirmed the increase in goblet cell numbers in cartilaginous airways in COPD [170, 572, 573]. In non-cartilaginous peripheral airways of internal diameter <2 mm, goblet cell numbers are increased ~3-fold in COPD [574]. Consistent with an increase in goblet cell numbers, immunocytochemistry has shown that MUC5AC in bronchiolar epithelium is increased in COPD, but MUC5B levels are not [575]. The numbers of a variety of inflammatory cells increase in the epithelium of small airways in chronic bronchitis [574].

The Reid Index increases from 0.26 to 0.4 in "healthy" controls to 0.50–0.60 in COPD [576], an average increase of ~1.5-fold (range = 1.2- to 2.1-fold). Using the relationship given in Section 1.4.1, the increases in Reid Index are converted to increases in *gland volume* of 1.3- to 3.9-fold (mean = 2.1-fold). All measurements of Reid Index have been made on samples obtained at necropsy, usually following death in hospital. In most studies, therefore, the control groups probably had some degree of unreported bronchitis [559]. Thus, the increase in total gland volume seen in going from a perfectly healthy to a badly diseased lung may be closer to the maximal calculated increase (3.9-fold) than the minimal (1.3-fold).

In chronic bronchitis, the smaller the airway the greater the relative increase in total gland volume. Thus, the total area of glands in conventional histological cross-sections is ~40% greater than normal in the trachea, ~two-fold greater in the main bronchi, and ~three-fold greater in segmental bronchi [557].

Whether, in chronic bronchitis, gland volume increases by hyperplasia or hypertrophy is unclear. In conventional cross sections of airway wall, it was early found that the cross-sectional area of individual mucous tubule profiles increased on average by 2.1-fold in COPD, while the area of individual serous profiles increased by 1.6-fold [577]. However, the overall thickness of the gland layer increased by 2.9-fold [577]. These results therefore suggest that the increase in total gland volume in chronic bronchitis is due both to hypertrophy (possibly due to distension of cells with mucus) and hyperplasia. Later studies emphasized the relative importance of hyperplasia. For instance, in studies on coal miners with COPD, the numbers of acini and tubules for a given area of gland tissue remained unchanged as the volume percent of gland profiles increased from 5% to 40% [578]. Whether this hyperplasia represents the formation of new tubules on pre-existing glands or the formation of entirely new glands is unclear.

Earlier anecdotal reports of an increase in the numbers of mucous gland profiles relative to serous in chronic bronchitis were tested quantitatively by de Haller and Reid [577]. They found that in healthy airways a microscopical field of the gland layer contained an average of 7 cross sectional profiles of mucous tubules and 8 of serous. By contrast, in chronic bronchitis a field of the same size contained on average 7 mucous profiles and 2 serous, a significantly different ratio of mucous to serous cells. Others, however, found that mucous cells accounted for 48% of gland volume in bronchitics and 41% in healthy controls, a difference that was not statistically significant [579].

The ratio of MUC5B to MUC5AC in sputum collected from patients with COPD ranges from 0.02 to 20, and is not statistically different from that for saline-induced sputum from healthy subjects [580]. However, in the *gel phase* of sputum, the ratio of MU5B/MUC5AC is significantly increased (by ~4-fold) in patients with COPD as compared with smokers without COPD. Further there is a significant negative correlation between the MUC5B/MUC5AC ratio and FEV_1/FVC [581]. These results strongly suggest that increased gland secretion plays an important role in the pathogenesis of COPD.

By contrast, another recent study [170] points to the primary importance of goblet cell secretions. First, there was a significant positive correlation between the number of pack-years and MUC5AC expression in surface epithelium. Second, there was a significant negative correlation between FEV_1 and surface epithelial MUC5AC levels. These relationships are hard to reconcile with the finding of others that MUC5AC levels in the gel phase of sputum from smokers are significantly reduced in COPD [580]. Another mildly surprising finding was the absence of changes in Reid Index or total gland area in COPD. However, half the COPD patients studied had emphysema but not chronic bronchitis, and changes in gland volume are much less in the former than the latter [560]. It is also notable that the Reid Index for healthy controls reported in this study (0.62) is somewhat greater than most earlier authors reported for chronic bronchitis! Interestingly, the total area of gland acini staining positively for MUC5AC (expressed as medians) increased from 2% in non-smokers to 9.5% in smokers without COPD to 20% in patients with COPD. The corresponding values for the area of gland occupied by MUC5B were 62%, 91% and 83% [170].

Subjects with COPD show histological evidence of inflammation around glands and gland ducts [582]. There are reports that the numbers of mast cells, neutrophils, macrophages, $CD45^+$ lymphocytes and plasma cells in airway glands are increased in chronic bronchitis [583–585]. The numbers of eosinophils do not change [585]. The numbers of gland-associated neutrophils correlates negatively with FEV_1 [585]. There may also be disease-related increases in nerve supply or neuronal tone to the glands [586, 587]. Thus, airway plugging in COPD is probably more dependent on stimulation of gland secretion by inflammatory mediators than on gland hypertrophy itself.

4.3   ASTHMA

Airway plugging with viscid mucus has long been recognized as a common pathological feature of deaths from asthma [561]. It is probable that >90% of airways in control subjects lack mucus plugs, whereas >90% of airways in fatal asthma are plugged to some degree [588]. MOR depends on the severity of the disease, with reported values for fatal asthma ranging from 10% to 60% [589–591]. Cells accounted for 66% of plug volume in airways of <3 mm luminal perimeter, but only ~33% in airways >12 mm in perimeter. In patients dying during long-term hospitalization for severe asthma, those that died from an acute asthma attack had higher MOR than those that died from other causes [592].

MOR shows no dependence on airway size for luminal perimeters between 2 mm to 20 mm [588]. This means that the ratio of mucus volume to airway surface area is about ten-fold greater in large glandular airways than small gland-free airways. The number of goblet cells is similar in large and small airways, so the increased secretory volume in the large airways presumably reflects gland secretion. In mucous plugs obtained with forceps from cross-sectional profiles of airways of a patient dying from asthma, MUC5B and MUC5AC accounted for ~86% and ~14%, respectively, of the total mucins [593], again consistent with an important contribution of glands to mucus accumulation in this disease.

In non-fatal asthma, gland volume have been reported as being unaltered [589, 594] or increased by ~50% [590]. This is consistent with an earlier report that gland volume in non-fatal asthma is much less than in chronic bronchitis [595]. In severe or fatal asthma, the increase in gland volume has been reported as two-fold [589, 590] or 4-fold over normal [591]. Somewhat surprisingly, of the various gland cell types, myoepithelial cells show the greatest relative increase in volume [590]. Echoing the findings for chronic bronchitis, the relative increase in gland volume in fatal asthma is greater in airways of 4–10 mm diameter than in those with diameters of 10–18 mm or >18 mm [594].

As in COPD, it may not be the overall size of the glands but rather their level of stimulation that is key to mucus secretion and airway plugging in asthma. Thus, as shown in Figure 30, whether in healthy controls, patients with non-fatal asthma, or those with fatal asthma, the MOR correlates significantly with the numbers of mast cells in the mucous glands [589]. Further, in fatal asthma, ~90% of gland-associated mast cells are degranulated as opposed to 45% in healthy airways, and there is a significant correlation between MOR and degranulated mast cells when data from fatal and non-fatal asthma are combined. Finally, though glands contained many fewer neutrophils than mast cells, the numbers of neutrophils per gland was also significantly elevated in asthma.

In mild to moderate asthma, goblet cell numbers in the main bronchi are doubled, and their aggregate volume tripled [596]. In patients dying of asthma attacks, the percentage of the epithelium occupied by goblet cells increased to ~50% from a control value of ~2.5% [591]. An interesting

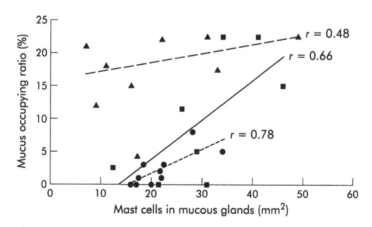

FIGURE 30: Dependence of mucus-plugging on the numbers of mast cells in airway glands. Triangles—fatal asthma; Squares—non-fatal asthma; Circles—controls. Lines are best least squared regressions for the three data sets. Taken from ref. [589].

finding of this study was that in asthma a large percentage of the luminal mucus remained in contact with mucus in goblet cells, though the same was not true of chronic bronchitis [591]. This will presumably hinder mucociliary clearance and contribute to mucus plugging in asthma.

The relative contributions of mucus plugging, smooth muscle contraction, and wall thickening to airflow obstruction in asthma are not precisely known. However, specific inhibition of mucin secretion greatly attenuates methacholine-induced increases in airway resistance in a mouse model of asthma [597].

Early studies pointed to abnormally high levels of airway epithelial desquamation in asthma with sheets of cells appearing in the lumen as so-called Creola bodies [598–600]. Furthermore, the numbers of epithelial cells in bronchoalveolar lavage fluid was reported as correlating with the severity of asthma [601, 602]. More recent work, however, has cast doubt on the possibility that epithelial shedding is increased in this disease [603].

In mild asthma, there is no change in nasal pd or in its responses to agents that alter active Na^+ absorption or Cl^- secretion [604] suggesting that barrier function (and ion transport) are normal. However, in more severe disease, the permeability of bronchial epithelium to the extracellular marker, DTPA, is markedly increased [605]. Further, compared to patients with cystic fibrosis or chronic bronchitis, asthmatics have greatly elevated levels of blood proteins in the tracheobronchial lumen [606]. By preventing protease-mediated mucus degradation, these plasma proteins may account for the peculiar rubbery quality of mucus plugs formed during acute asthma attacks [607]. Thus, epithelial barrier function may be compromised more in asthma than in cystic fibrosis or chronic bronchitis.

It has generally been thought that the changes in airway epithelial function in asthma were caused by inflammation. However, it has recently been proposed that the airway epithelium plays a "sentinel role" in asthma with intrinsic changes in epithelial function underlying most of the pathology of the disease [554]. The evidence for this new view comes largely from work on primary cultures of human airway epithelium. The cultures are initiated from brushings, and generally used after two to five passages. Cells are often grown on Petri dishes, though occasionally on inserts with an air–liquid interface. In a substantial number of these papers, the details of the culture procedures are very scanty, and little attempt is made to describe the overall level of differentiation of the cultured cells. This is unfortunate, as it is possible that some of the abnormalities ascribed to asthma are in fact culture artifacts. One major problem is that the cellular composition of airway surface epithelium is altered in asthma, and the composition of the cell suspensions used to initiate the primary cultures will likewise be altered. Different attachment efficiencies will result that, in turn, will influence the final phenotype of the confluent cell sheets. Thus, high levels of attachment produce relatively columnar and well-differentiated confluent cell sheets. At lower levels, it takes longer for the cell cultures to reach confluence and the resulting cell sheets tend to be much more squamous and less differentiated, changes reflected in lower I_{sc} [306]. Furthermore, these differences in phenotype are likely to persist even with repeated passaging; a dispersion of columnar cells is likely to have a different attachment efficiency and rate of division than is a dispersion of squamous cells. A second problem is that the effects of inflammation can persist for weeks in culture [608]. A third problem is that the culture conditions used have often been sub-optimal, and an intrinsic asthma-related difference expressed in undifferentiated cultures may not apply to native epithelium. A dramatic example of how differentiation can affect results is the finding that poorly differentiated squamous cultures of human tracheal epithelium show levels of rhinoviral infection some 1000-fold greater than do well-differentiated cultures of mucociliary phenotype [609].

The best approach to obtaining well-differentiated cultures is to plate at high densities on porous-bottomed inserts with air-interface feeding; the resulting cultures may be virtually indistinguishable, structurally and functionally, from native epithelium [306, 610]. By contrast, low plating densities, growth on solid supports, and immersion feeding all tend to produce highly squamous undifferentiated cultures [306, 611]. Even at high plating densities, cells grown on solid supports may fail to form tight junctions and polarize [611]. Repeated passaging also promotes dedifferentiation, with the number of passages that can be achieved without marked dedifferentiation often being no more than two [612–614]. Finally, the choice of culture medium is critically important [615]. Because of the extreme variability in levels of differentiation obtained in culture, a detailed description of the culture methods is imperative. And, second, a careful comparison should be made of several markers of differentiation in the cells derived from asthmatics vs. non-asthmatics. Measurements of DNA and total cell protein, as estimates of cell number and cell sheet height, respectively, have the advantage over histology in that they are quantitative and less subject to investigator bias. Measures of R_{te} establish whether or not the cells have formed tight junctions and polarized.

Because the culture conditions used can markedly affect the results obtained, and because lack of characterization of cells can cast doubt on the validity of the conclusions, in the following descriptions of work done with airway epithelial cultures derived from asthmatics, brief descriptions of the culture approaches used and of the phenotypes obtained are included.

Cells were obtained from brushings and passaged 2 or 3 times. They were grown in "culture dishes," and passaged 2 or 3 times. There were "no gross morphological" differences between normal and asthmatic cultures [616]. The cells were later shown to have a basal cell phenotype in that they stained for cytokeratin 13 [617]. The mean generation time of these cells was unaffected by asthma [616]. Cells from asthmatics showed no change in apoptosis under baseline conditions, but did show greater than control levels of apoptosis in the presence of H_2O_2, but not TNFα or actinomycin-D [616]. Native airway epithelium was also shown to have increased levels of apoptosis in asthma [616]. Cells from asthmatics had increased expression of p21 (waf) cyclin-dependent kinase inhibitor [618], increased release of TGFα in response to either TNFα or combinations of IL-4, IL-13, and Der p [619], and a deficient innate immune response to rhinovirus [617].

Passage 2 cells grown with an air-liquid interface on porous-bottomed inserts for 21 days contained basal, ciliated and goblet cells as revealed by transmission electron microscopy. Cells from asthmatics showed marked disruption of ZO-1 staining and lower levels of ZO-1 protein expression. However, these gross structural and biochemical abnormalities had surprisingly little effect on R_{te}, which was unchanged by asthma at 7 and 14 days of culture, though at 21 days the median R_{te} was reduced from ~450 Ω cm^2 to ~350 Ω cm^2 (Figure 31A). At this time the permeability to 4 kDa and 20 kDa dextrans was also increased (significantly) by ~2-fold over control in asthma. Significant changes in R_{te} or dextran fluxes were only seen in cells from patients with severe asthma, not in mild or moderate asthma. The drop in R_{te} induced by cigarette smoke was significantly enhanced in asthma, and cells from asthmatics, but not controls, showed a small but significant increase in R_{te} in response to EGF [620]. In another study [621], cells were grown in T$_{75}$ flasks until 80% confluent, and then passaged at 0.8×10^5 cells/Transwell, where they grew to confluence in 5 to 7 days. The level of mucociliary differentiation as revealed by conventional transmission electron microscopy was excellent. There were no differences in total cell number in cultures from asthmatics, but there were significantly more goblet cells and fewer ciliated cells. However, there were no asthma-related changes in R_{te} from 7 to 28 days after attaining confluence (Figure 31B). Nor did asthma affect the release of IL-8, IL-6 or PGE$_2$ [621].

Epithelium was microdissected from airways obtained at lobectomy or pulmonectomy and grown in explant culture on Petri dishes for 2–3 weeks, by which time the outgrowth of cells had

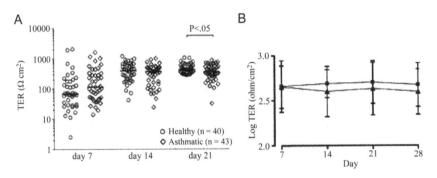

FIGURE 31: Effects of asthma on R_{te} of passaged primary cultures of human tracheal epithelium. A) R_{te} at various times following plating. Horizontal bars are medians. Taken from ref. [620]. B) R_{te} at various times following attainment of confluency. Values are means ± SD, $n = 7$ for asthmatics (triangles) or $n = 9$ for controls (squares). Taken from ref. [621].

become confluent [622]. The baseline ciliary beat frequency was not significantly altered by asthma. Nor was its inhibition by diesel exhaust particles. However, asthma significantly increased the constitutive release of IL-8, GM-CSF, sICAM-1 and RANTES. Stimulation of release of these mediators by diesel exhaust particles was also enhanced [622, 623]. In further studies, explants were used to generate confluent outgrowths on Petri dishes. The explants were then removed and placed on inserts, where they again produced confluent cell sheets [624]. Asthma did not alter the constitutive release of IL-8, GM-CSF and sICAM-1 from these cultures. At one of three doses of ozone, GM-CSF and sICAM1, but not IL-8, showed enhanced release in asthma [624]. Releases stimulated by NO_2 were unaltered in asthma.

Epithelial cells were expanded in T_{75} flasks and then trypsinized and plated onto inserts, where they developed ciliated and goblet cells. Cultures from patients with severe asthma produced more mucin and IL-8, but less lipoxinA4, than did cells from patients with mild asthma. Expression of MUC5AC, MUC5B, 5-LPO or 15-LPO was not affected by the severity of the asthma [625].

Cells from asthmatics, grown in Petri dishes and passaged up to five times, proliferated about twice as fast as normal [626]. They released 25 times as much IL-6, 3 times as much PGE_2, twice as much EGF, but only one third as much TBFβ-1; release of IL-1β, sICAM-1 and IL-8 was unchanged. This release profile was maintained through successive passages [626]. When cells were scraped off, the recolonization of the denuded area was slowed in asthma, an effect related to impaired ability to synthesize fibronectin [627].

Normal and asthmatic primary cultures grown on inserts were obtained from a commercial vendor. After wounding, the cells from asthmatics showed greater than normal production of TGFβ-1, IL-10, IL-13 and IL-1β, but not IL-6. They divided less and regenerated the wounded area less rapidly [628].

To summarize these cell culture studies: 1) Measurements of R_{te} indicate that intrinsic changes in barrier function in asthma are quite subtle, and only seen in severe disease; however, culture artifacts will be more prevalent in cultures from patients with severe disease. 2) Changes in release of inflammatory mediators in asthma are not dramatic. Many studies find no changes. Others detect small changes in response to a limited number of specific stimuli. 3) Two studies have reported reduced wound healing in asthma.

4.4 CYSTIC FIBROSIS
4.4.1 Gross Pathology
Cystic fibrosis is a genetic disease caused by mutations in the gene coding for the cystic fibrosis transmembrane conductance regulator (CFTR), a cAMP-activated Cl^- channel found mainly in epithelia. Many organs are affected, and in most the pathology is associated with excessively dry mucus. Death usually results from the consequences of bacterial colonization of the airways [629,

630]. Changes in the ASL that promote this colonization may include increased acidity [286], reduced secretion of antimicrobials [522, 631], altered salt content [462], or failure of mucociliary clearance due to collapse of the periciliary sol [465] or increased viscosity of the gel [469]. Bacterial colonization sets in motion a viscous inflammatory cascade. Massive numbers of neutrophils migrate into the airways to kill the bacteria [551], which promptly protect themselves by secreting gelatinous coats [632]. Transepithelial migration of neutrophils [551] and inflammatory mediators stimulate mucus secretion and plasma transudation. Over time hypertrophy of the airway glands [556, 633] and mucous metaplasia of the surface epithelium develop [633] resulting in still more mucus. DNA from dead leukocytes binds together mucus, jelly, bugs, plasma proteins and cell debris [634]. Bronchiectasis virtually always ensues [633].

In children dying of CF in the first 4 months of life, approximately two-thirds of all airways showed some degree of mucopurulent plugging. By the age of 6 years, plugs were present in all airways [633]. In a recent study [635] of non-cartilaginous airways (bronchioles) obtained at transplantation, mucous plugs occupied on average more than 50% of the luminal area of airway cross sections in CF and the epithelium showed dramatic mucous metaplasia (Figure 32). Further there was a many-fold increase in the numbers of neutrophils per unit area of epithelial surface (Figure 32). There was a negative correlation between the amount of mucin in the epithelium and the numbers of neutrophils in the lumen, suggesting that neutrophils were stimulating mucin release. Consistent with bronchiectasis, the airway diameters were 3-fold greater than normal in

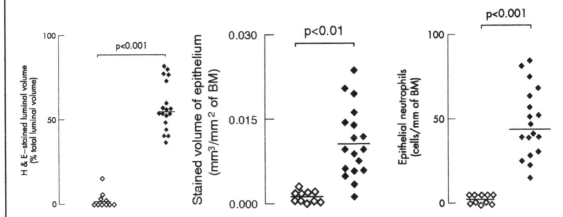

FIGURE 32: Changes in structure of small airways in CF. Mucus in the airway lumen was determined by staining with hematoxylin and eosin and expressed as the mucus-occupying ratio (left panel). Mucins in the epithelium (expressed as stained volume) were determined by PAS/Alcian blue staining (middle panel). Numbers of neutrophils within the epithelium were measured in cross sections and normalized to the length of basemant membrane (right panel). Open symbols—non-CF; closed symbols—CF. Taken from ref. [635].

CF (0.6 vs. 2.0 mm). An interesting feature of this study was that in CF the volume of epithelium staining for MUC5B was approximately equal to the volume staining for MUC5AC. Similar levels of the two mucins were also found in the mucous plugs [635]. Others have reported that the basic distributions of mucins are unchanged in CF airways: MUC5AC remains the predominant mucin of goblet cells, MUC5B of glands [169].

In large (cartilaginous) airways, the bronchial surface epithelium shows regions of both squamous and mucous metaplasia in CF that increase in frequency with age [629, 633]. However, a recent stereological analysis failed to find a significant change in the number of goblet cells per unit area of basement membrane of cartilaginous airways, though there was a significant 50% increase in the average volume of the goblet cells [556]. In the CF pig, the epithelium of large airways also shows focal goblet cell hyperplasia [636].

Gland hypertrophy in CF was early recognized [637], and the Reid index is increased significantly [633, 638]. Interestingly, in one study [633], the Index showed no dependence on age in CF, being the same in patients dying within 14 days of birth as in adults. However, others have failed to confirm gland hypertrophy in children less than one year old [639, 640]. Most recently, in second to fourth generation airways gland volume per unit area of surface (as determined by stereology) has been shown to increase by 2.8-fold in CF [556].

4.4.2   Overview of CF-Related Defects

What intrinsic changes in the function of airway epithelium trigger the airway pathology of CF? Table 6 provides a reasonably complete list of the bewildering array of possibilities that have been advanced. These can be divided into five basic categories: failure of CFTR channel function; interactions of CFTR with other channels; hyperinflammatory changes, developmental changes, and miscellaneous. The list of airway epithelial functions that have been definitively shown to be unaltered in CF is much shorter (see Table 7).

In the sections that follow, the established and putative intrinsic defects in CF will be treated in approximately the same order as listed in Table 6. Lack of Cl^- secretion and elevated Na^+ absorption, however, will be dealt with together as these two defects should have synergistic effects on mucociliary clearance. Emphasis will be placed on those defects that are most likely to alter mucociliary clearance or the concentrations of antimicrobials in ASL, but references will be provided for other proposed defects.

4.4.3   Reduced Bicarbonate Secretion

Bicarbonate secretion plays an important role in airway gland liquid secretions (Section 3). The route for HCO_3^- efflux across the apical membrane of gland serous cells is CaCC with cholinergic stimulation, and CFTR with cAMP-dependent stimulation [519]. It was therefore unsurprising

TABLE 6: Intrinsic changes in airway epithelial function in CF.
SOME ESTABLISHED DEFECTS IN CFTR CHANNEL ACTIVITY AND THEIR POTENTIAL CONSEQUENCES
Lack of cAMP-dependent Cl$^-$ secretion in glands
Viscous gland secretions
Less antimicrobials secreted
Lack of cAMP-dependent Cl$^-$ conductance in surface epithelium
Increased viscosity of mucus blanket
Depletion of the periciliary sol
Reduced NaCl concentration in ASL (and therefore reduced antimicrobial activity)
Lack of HCO$_3^-$ secretion in surface and gland epithelia
Acidic ASL & compromised antimicrobial activity
Reduced expansion of mucus on release
Lack of SCN$^-$ secretion by surface epithelium
Reduced antimicrobial activity
Lack of glutathione secretion
Reduced protection from oxidant damage
SOME CONTROVERSIAL DEFECTS IN CFTR CHANNEL ACTIVITY AND THEIR POTENTIAL CONSEQUENCES
Lack of CFTR channel function in intracellular organelles
Multiple effects including altered sulfation and glycosylation of mucins
Lack of ATP secretion
Multiple effects on mucociliary clearance

TABLE 6: (continued)
SOME CF-RELATED EFFECTS ON OTHER MEMBRANE TRANSPORT PROCESSES
Elevated active Na^+ absorption
Depletion of periciliary sol and increased viscosity of mucous gel
Induction of cAMP-dependence on the ORDIC Cl^- channel
Upregulation of CaCC and SCL26A9 and downregulation of volume-activated Cl^- channels
Altered function of K^+ channels
Inhibition of aquaporin-3
Inhibition of Cl^-/HCO_3^- exchange and stimulation of Na^+/H^+ exchange
HYPERINFLAMMATORY CHANGES
Increased cytokine release/increased activation of NFkB
Increased Pseudomonas binding
Decreased Pseudomonas binding
Decreased NO production
Compromised wound healing
Altered STAT pathways
Enhanced intracellular Ca signaling
Decreased apoptosis
Reduced smad3 signaling
DEVELOPMENTAL CHANGES
More glands
Smaller glands
Altered stem cell niches

TABLE 6: *(continued)*
OTHER CHANGES
Lack of cAMP-mediated gap junctional communication
Abnormal secretory granules in glands
Elevated activity of lysosomal enzymes
Hypersecretion of serous cell antimicrobials
Inhibition of endocytosis and stimulation of exocytosis
Altered interactions with trafficking proteins
Defective glycoconjugate secretion
Increased paracellular permeability
Decreased interaction with protein kinase CK2
Impaired cholesterol trafficking
Decreased AMPK activity

TABLE 7: Airway epithelial functions that are unaltered in CF.
Protein kinase A activity [641]
Mucus granule release from surface epithelial goblet cells [71]
Transepithelial neutrophil migration [642]
Osmotic water permeability [132]

that fluorescent probes injected into carbachol-induced tracheal gland secretions showed that their pH was unchanged in CF from the normal value of ~6.95 [526]. However, in a second study from the same group, normal nasal gland secretions, induced again with carbachol, had pH 7.18; those from CF patients were significantly lower at 6.57. Further, CFTR inhibitors reduced the pH of normal gland secretions to about the same value as seen in CF glands [288]. In the first study specimens were obtained at the time of lung transplantation; in the second, nasal biopsies were obtained from relatively young patients undergoing otolaryngological procedures.

Given that CFTR transports HCO_3^- [643], ASL in CF would be expected to be abnormally acidic. One early study provided support for this hypothesis. The surface of primary cultures of human bronchial epithelium was covered with 100 μl of unbuffered saline. Samples were then withdrawn at set intervals, equilibrated with 5% CO_2 and their pH determined. The pH of the samples taken from CF cells approached an asymptotic value of ~6, whereas normal cells approached a value of ~6.25 [289]. Others, using pH probes (tip diameter of 1 to 2 mm) failed to detect a significant difference in the pH of nasal ASL in CF in vivo [644]. In tracheas of CF mice, fluorescent probes failed to find altered ASL pH [341]. However, in mouse trachea, CaCC makes an overwhelmingly greater contribution to apical membrane Cl^- conductance than does CFTR [645]. In the newborn CF pig in vivo, pH-sensitive foil was placed directly on the tracheal surface and the signal measured with an optical probe. To measure pH over cultures, 200 μl of perfluorocarbon containing a pH-sensitive probe was placed on the mucosal surface and fluorescence intensity measured 2 h later. Both approaches showed that ASL pH was more acidic in porcine CF, by 0.3 pH units in native epithelium and 0.4 in cultures [286]. Further, the CF ASL was less effective at killing bacteria than the non-CF. This was not due to differences in the concentrations of either the major endogenous antimicrobials or of Na^+ and Cl^-. However, reducing ASL pH diminished bacterial killing in wild-type pigs, and increasing ASL pH rescued killing in CF pigs [286]. Thus, increased acidity of airway ASL in CF may inhibit endogenous antimicrobial function and thereby contribute to bacterial colonization.

Bicarbonate transport across freshly excised nasal tissue has recently been measured by pH stat [646]. The rate of HCO_3^- secretion was reduced by 80% in CF. Furthermore, the equilibrium pH attained in the unbuffered mucosal medium was significantly more acidic in CF.

Mucins are stored in highly condensed form in intracellular granules by shielding of their cationic sites with H^+ or cross-linking of them with Ca^{2+} [175]. It has been proposed that by reacting with the H^+ and Ca^{2+}, HCO_3^- facilitates the expansion of mucin granules following their exocytosis. It is assumed that the HCO_3^- involved is extracellular. Therefore, with the reduced HCO_3^- levels in ASL in CF, mucins will not hydrate and expand to the normal extent [555]. Support for this hypothesis has been obtained in the intestinal and uterine tracts [647, 648]. For instance, when female reproductive tracts of mice were mounted in bicarbonate-buffered physiological saline, and their lumens perfused, a combination of PGE_2 and carbachol caused mucus to appear in the perfusate. This mucus secretion was absent in the CF mouse, in normal mice when serosal HCO_3^- was removed, or in normal mice when HCO_3^- secretion had been blocked pharmacologically. Histology indicated that with reduced levels of luminal HCO_3^-, mucin exocytosis was normal. However, inadequate expansion of the mucus granules left the mucins attached to the cell surface rather than free in the perfusate [647].

4.4.4   Altered Gland Fluid Secretion

The surface of sheets of human trachea was covered with paraffin oil, under which beads of carbachol-induced secretions pooled up over individual gland openings. Small aliquots of dextran-FITC were injected into beads and allowed to equilibrate. A column of liquid within an individual bead was photo-bleached, and the rate of diffusion of dextran-FITC into the bleached area measured. In CF tissues, the rate of recovery of fluorescence was twice as slow as normal. It was concluded that gland secretions were abnormally viscous in CF [526]. This increase in viscosity was consistent with findings from the same group that cholinergically induced fluid flows from nasal glands were reduced by ~60% in CF [649], and that a specific CFTR inhibitor decreased cholinergically mediated fluid flow from non-CF airway glands by ~60% [650].

The finding of increased viscosity of carbachol-induced secretions, however, is puzzling in the light of other work indicating that cholinergically mediated fluid flows from glands are mediated almost entirely by CaCC, with very little contribution from CFTR. The evidence for this is as follows. First, using the same technique for measuring gland flows, a separate group found that cholinergically mediated fluid secretion by tracheal airway glands was unaltered in CF [524]. This discrepancy could be explained by the fact that the nasal biopsies used in the measurements of mucus viscosity were taken from young CF subjects with minimal clinical disease. However, second, cholinergically mediated fluid flows across cultures of human tracheal gland epithelium are unaltered in CF [651]. Third, the shrinkage of pig serous cell acini (i.e., Cl^- secretion) induced by carbachol is unaffected by blockers of CFTR, but is inhibited by blockers of CaCC [517]. One possible explanation for increased viscosity of carbachol-induced gland secretions in CF is that baseline CFTR-dependent gland liquid secretion is lacking in CF [522]. Therefore, mucins may build up in the duct lumens. This accumulated mucus will be flushed out on cholinergic stimulation and could account for the increased viscosity of gland secretions in CF. If this is so, then the viscosity should decline with increased duration of exposure to cholinergic agents.

Recently, Martens et al. [545] have collected aggregate secretions from non-CF and CF human bronchi following stimulation with a variety of mediators. They found that for any given flow rate, the CF secretions were about twice as concentrated as normal. An unusual aspect of this study, however, is that forskolin induced secretions in CF bronchi, but others have shown that CF glands do not respond to this or any other agent that acts through cAMP [498, 522, 652].

Non-CF glands secrete fluid in response to elevation of cAMP. Further, there is synergy between cAMP- and Ca-elevating agents in non-CF glands that is absent in CF. Thus, as shown in Figure 33A, doses of carbachol and VIP that had no effect in themselves, when combined stimulated secretion. The mechanism of this synergy is simple. Low levels of carbachol activate basolateral K^+ channels but not apical membrane CaCC. Low doses of VIP activate CFTR but not basolateral K$^+$ channels. Activation of both apical Cl$^-$ channels and basolateral K$^+$ channels is required for Cl$^-$ secretion. In CF, there was no response to either or both agents (Figure 33B), though the tissues were viable as indicated by robust responses to high doses of cholinergic agents delivered at the end of the experiment.

These results led to the hypothesis that low levels of acetylcholine and VIP release under baseline condition in vivo stimulate a low level of resting gland secretion that is CFTR-dependent. Lack of this baseline fluid secretion in CF would reduce the amount of gland antimicrobials reaching the surface, and therefore promote bacterial colonization. In cats, baseline gland secretion in vivo is about half the level of maximal cholinergically induced gland secretion [30]. In dogs, baseline secretion is ~30% that induced by Substance P [653].

It has recently been shown that the cytokines, IL-1β and TNF-α stimulate CFTR-mediated fluid secretion from pig airway glands [654]. The significance of this is that both cytokines are released by Pseudomonas infection of the airways, and lack of this bacterially induced flushing action should also promote bacterial colonization in CF.

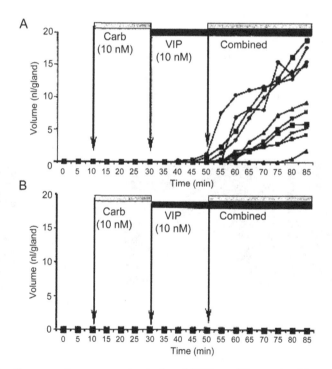

FIGURE 33: Lack of synergy between carbachol and VIP in CF glands. A) Normal glands. B) CF glands ($n = 10$). Taken from ref. [524].

4.4.5 Airway Surface Epithelial Ion Transport and Failure of Mucociliary Clearance in CF

In primary cultures of human nasal or tracheal epithelium from subjects without CF, mucus is transported in a circular fashion around the center of the cell sheet (Figure 34). By contrast, mucus in CF cultures is essentially static (Figure 34) [461]. It was proposed that this failure of mucus transport in CF was due not only to a lack of cAMP-dependent Cl^- secretion but also to elevated active Na^+ absorption. The increased liquid absorption caused by this combination of changes then led to a collapse of the periciliary sol and condensation of the mucous gel. With less room for the cilia to beat, and a more viscous gel for them to propel, mucous transport failed. Several papers from the group that proposed this hypothesis showed a significant decrease in the depth of ASL in CF of ~33% some 24 to 48 h after adding 100 μl of PBS to the mucosal surface of 1 cm^2 (for an average increase in ASL depth of 1 mm) [455, 465]. The PBS was added in order to deliver a fluorescent marker of the ASL; at the rate of fluid absorption of 5 μl cm^{-2} h^{-1} reported by others [32], the ASL should have returned to its original volume within 20 h. This group, however, reports fluid absorption across their cultures of 0.7 μl cm^{-2} h^{-1} [130].

What is the evidence for elevated active Na^+ absorption in CF? In 1981 [304] it was reported that the nasal pd was doubled in CF and showed increased sensitivity to superfusion of amiloride (Figure 35A). This result has been repeatedly confirmed, and nasal pd measurements are now used diagnostically in CF, particularly in cases with borderline or normal sweat tests. Shortly afterwards, it was shown that the I_{sc} of cultures of human nasal epithelium was similarly doubled in CF and also

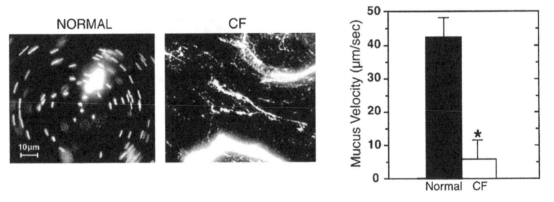

FIGURE 34: Failure of mucociliary transport in CF. Long exposure (5 s) micrographs of fluorescent beads added to the surface of airway epithelial cultures. The normal culture exhibited movement of beads around the center; the CF culture demonstrated clumps of beads that did not move. The mean velocities for the beads on normal and CF cultures are shown in the right panel (*$P < 0.05$, compared to normal; n = six per group). Taken from ref. [461].

A

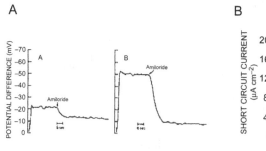

B

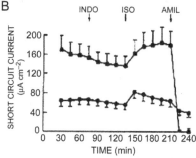

FIGURE 35: Increased active Na$^+$ absorption in CF. A) Effects of amiloride on nasal pd in CF patients (right panel) and non-CF controls (left panel). Taken from ref. [655]. B) I_{sc} across primary cultures of human tracheal epithelium. Squares—CF; Circles—non-CF. INDO—indomethacin; ISO—isoproterenol; AMIL—amiloride. Taken from ref. [314].

showed increased sensitivity to amiloride (Figure 35B). Further, measurements of transepithelial ^{22}Na fluxes showed that the doubling of I_{sc} in CF was entirely accountable for by increased net absorption of Na$^+$ [314]. Finally, when CFTR and ENaC were co-expressed in MDCK cells or fibroblasts, CFTR inhibited ENaC [656], though this effect could not be seen in Xenopus oocytes [657].

By what means is Na$^+$ absorption elevated in CF? An early report of increased NaKATPase levels in airway epithelium in CF [658] has not been independently confirmed. The levels of mRNA for the various subunits of ENaC are unaltered in airway epithelium [370]. However, it has been proposed that wild-type CFTR decreases trafficking of ENaC to the apical membrane [659]. It has also been suggested that the probability of opening (P_o) of ENaC is somehow increased in CF. Several potential mechanisms have been advanced. First, the presence of wild-type CFTR converts the action of PKA on P_o of ENaC from stimulatory to inhibitory [660]. Second, direct physical interaction between CFTR and ENaC [661, 662] protects ENaC from cleavage and activation by proteolysis [662]. Third, the inhibitory interaction may be via actin [663]. Fourth, prostasin expression is increased by 50% in CF [234] leading to greater cleavage and activation of ENaC. However, SPLUNC levels are increased in ASL in CF and this should reduce the activation of ENaC by preventing proteolysis [664].

Consistent with the increase in active Na$^+$ absorption, we reported that fluid absorption was doubled across cultures of nasal epithelium in CF, and increased by ~50% across tracheal cultures [32].

Recent work from Michael Welsh's group [470, 665], however, convincingly shows that 1) airway ENaC activity is not altered in CF, 2) the increased Na$^+$ absorption under short-circuit conditions can be accounted for entirely by a lack of the CFTR Cl$^-$ conductance in the apical membrane, 3) net absorption of salts and water is not increased in CF under open-circuit conditions, 4) there is no change in the depth of ASL in CF.

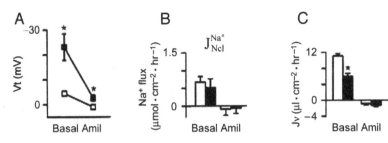

FIGURE 36: Transport of salt and water across nasal epithelium in CF pigs. A) Nasal pd is elevated in CF. B) Open-circuit net Na^+ absorption is unaltered in CF. C) Open-circuit water absorption is decreased in CF. All these parameters are abolished, or nearly so, by amiloride (AMIL). *—significantly different from corresponding non-CF value. Open symbols—non-CF; closed symbols—CF. Means ± SE. Taken from ref. [470].

In newborn CF pigs, the nasal pd was elevated and showed increased sensitivity to amiloride (Figure 36A). Furthermore, baseline I_{sc} across nasal epithelium was also significantly elevated. However, under open-circuit conditions, net Na^+ absorption was unchanged (Figure 36B), and net liquid absorption was even somewhat reduced (Figure 36C) [470].

V_{te} and I_{sc} of non-CF nasal epithelium were negatively correlated with the apical membrane Cl conductance. In other words, the increases in V_{te} and I_{sc} in CF were due to changes in V_a consequent on reduced apical membrane Cl^- conductance. In a key experiment, replacement of Cl^- with the impermeant gluconate$^-$ caused V_{te} and I_{sc} of non-CF nasal cultures to become identical to those of CF cultures. This argues strongly that the apical membrane Na^+ conductance is unaltered in CF.

Similar results were obtained on pig and human tracheas: net open-circuit absorption of Na^+ and water was unaltered in CF [470, 665]. Nor, in pig trachea in vivo, was the depth of ASL changed in CF [470]. The trachea, however, differed from the nose in that its V_{te} and I_{sc} were not elevated in CF, a difference ascribed to a lower apical membrane CFTR-mediated Cl^- conductance than in nasal epithelium.

Evidence from other groups also argues against increased ENaC activity leading to depletion of ASL volume in CF. First, others have found that net open-circuit absorption of Na^+ across nasal epithelium is unaltered in CF [333, 666]. Second, equivalent circuit analysis readily shows that lack of an apical membrane Cl^- channel can increase V_{te} and I_{sc} and their sensitivity to amiloride without change in apical membrane Na^+ conductance [667, 668]. Third, the recent immunocytochemical finding that ENaC is found predominantly on cilia and CFTR on microvilli [68] makes regulation of ENaC by CFTR unlikely. Finally, a second group has independently confirmed using primary cultures of human tracheal epithelium that ASL depth is unaltered in CF [469].

If ASL depth is unaltered in CF, then what accounts for the reduced mucus transport in CF cultures? Recent data suggest that the viscosity of sol and gel in CF is increased by unknown mechanisms that are largely independent of transepithelial water flows. Powdered FITC-dextran was added to the ASL over primary cultures of human tracheal epithelium, and allowed to dissolve. There was thus no significant perturbation of ASL volume. Areas of mucus gel or periciliary sol were photobleached, and estimates of viscosity were made from the recovery of fluorescence over time. The baseline viscosity of both sol and gel was elevated 3- to 4-fold in CF [469]. These were cultures in which mucous secretions had accumulated for some time, and the depth of ASL was ~15 μm in both CF and non-CF cells. Thus, the difference in viscosity was not due to a difference in mucus concentration caused by a difference in volume. The other possibilities to explain the increased viscosity in CF are a higher mucus concentration due to more mucus secreted or less degraded, a difference in the types of mucins secreted in CF, or an altered balance of factors that affect mucus viscosity. Regarding the last, lack of HCO_3^- in ASL could increase mucus viscosity by hindering mucin granule expansion [555]. The finding that the viscosity of the periciliary sol is increased in CF is harder to explain. There are thought to be no gel-forming mucins in the periciliary sol, so the increase in viscosity is presumably due either to a greater abundance of the membrane-bound mucins, MUC1 and MUC4, or to a pH-dependent change in the interactions between their extracellular domains.

The effects on viscosity of agents expected to alter ASL volume are puzzling. In normal cultures neither amiloride nor forskolin affected viscosity. However, amiloride did not affect ASL depth significantly though forskolin increased it by 73% [467]. In CF cultures, forskolin had no effect on depth or viscosity. Amiloride increased depth by 70% (i.e., 1.7-fold) but decreased viscosity by 75% (i.e., 4-fold).

4.4.6 The High Salt Hypothesis

Bacteria added to the mucosal surface of highly differentiated, ciliated cultures were killed much less readily than normal in CF [669]. ASL was collected, and found to be less bactericidal in CF. Adding salt to the mucosal surface of normal cultures reduced their killing ability, adding water to the surface of CF cultures increased their killing ability. ASL collected from the nose in vivo suggested that its Cl^- concentration was increased from ~125 to ~175 mM in CF. It was hypothesized that CF ASL had reduced antimicrobial activity because it was saltier than normal; many endogenous antimicrobials work better when tonicity is reduced [235, 670, 671].

It was accordingly proposed that the ASL was held in place by surface tension, and that active Na^+ transport reduced its NaCl concentration to less than that of plasma. It was proposed that much of the Cl^- that followed the Na^+ took a CFTR-dependent transcellular route, and loss of this route in CF led to increased $[NaCl]_{ASL}$ and reduced antimicrobial activity [454]. However, recent measurements of NaCl content and osmolarity of ASL have provided little support for this theory; the osmolarity, $[Na^+]$ and $[Cl^-]$ of ASL are similar to those of plasma and not altered in CF or by CFTR inhibitors [286, 341, 463, 464].

4.4.7   Transport of Other Solutes Through CFTR

Lack of SCN^- secretion in primary cultures of CF airway epithelium leads to reduced ability to kill bacteria [631, 672]. However, samples (~20 μl total volume) of nasal ASL obtained in vivo showed no change in $[SCN^-]$ with CF in humans and only a drop of about 50% in pigs [673]. CFTR conducts SCN^-, but inflammation up-regulates CFTR-independent transport mechanisms. Thus, ATP induces SCN^- fluxes through CaCC that are some ten-fold higher than the CFTR-dependent fluxes [430]. Further, treatment with the inflammatory mediator, IL-4, induces pendrin-dependent Cl^-/SCN^- exchange that is again considerably higher than the baseline CFTR-dependent SCN^- flux [430].

   Glutathione, an anionic tripeptide, is the most important antioxidant in the lung [674]. Both reduced (GSH) and oxidized glutathione (GSSG) are transported by CFTR [278, 675] but only from the inside to the outside of the cell [278]. The permeability of CFTR to GSH is about one tenth that to Cl^-, and the permeability to GSSG about one hundredth [278]. GSH levels are reduced in CF ASL [676], though how much this is due to increased oxidant stress vs. reduced secretion is unclear. There are multiple ways that reduced levels of GSH will impact the airway pathology of CF. Interestingly, GSH has a mucolytic action, so its relative lack in CF could promote increased mucus viscosity [677].

   It has been proposed that CFTR conducts ATP and that the Mg–ATP complex has a planar diameter sufficiently small to penetrate the CFTR pore [678, 679]. This theory, however, has not met with general acceptance [680, 681]. Failure of CFTR to conduct ATP would influence mucociliary clearance by actions on mucin secretion, ciliary beat frequency, Cl^- secretion and Na^+ absorption.

4.4.8   Defective Organellar Acidification

The interior of intracellular organelles is invariably more acidic than that of cytosol—in the case of lysosomes by ~2.5 pH units. The primary mechanism for acidification of organelles is an H^+-ATPase. It was proposed that Cl^- flow through CFTR provided a counter anion to the actively transported protons. Therefore, in the absence of functioning CFTR, organelles would develop a larger transmembrane potential but their interiors would be less acidic [682]. The resulting change in the activity of Golgi enzymes could then account for early reports of decreased protein sialylation, increased fucosylation and sulfation, and increased numbers of asialo-gangliosides in CF [683]. These changes would contribute to CF pathology by altering the rheological properties of mucus, and by increasing Pseudomonas binding (asialo-gangliosides are putative Pseudomonas binding sites). In fact, decreased acidity of intracellular organelles could potentially account for every aspect of CF pathology. Unfortunately, many sophisticated approaches have shown that there are no alterations in vacuolar pH in CF [684, 685]. Nor are there any intrinsic CF-related alterations in glycosylation and sulfation of mucins [686–689]. Instead, any changes are likely due to inflammation, as indicated by the finding that COPD and CF share similar changes in the glycosylation of airway mucins [162].

4.4.9   Interactions of CFTR with Ion Channels/Transporters Other than ENaC

Shortly after the apical membrane of airway epithelium was shown to lack a Cl⁻ conductance [349, 690], patch-clamping of airway epithelial cells revealed a characteristic Cl⁻ channel that showed cAMP-dependent activation in normal cells but not CF [691, 692]. Expression studies, however, soon indicated that this outwardly rectifying depolarization-induced channel, or ORDIC [693], was not the defective Cl conductance in CF [694, 695]. It was, however, later reported that though ORDIC was indeed the wrong channel, the presence of CFTR somehow caused it to become sensitive to cAMP [696, 697].

Since then, CFTR has been shown to influence a large number of other channels. There is evidence that wild-type CFTR inhibits CaCC. Thus, superfusion of the nasal surface with ATP or UTP results in increases in nasal pd that are two-fold greater than normal in CF [698]. Similarly, in cultures of human nasal epithelium, the ATP-induced increase in apical membrane Cl⁻ permeability is twice normal in CF [398]. Calcium-mediated Cl⁻ secretion is also abnormally elevated in the nasal epithelium of CF mice [699]. Consistent with these findings, expression and activation of wild-type CFTR in CF cell lines inhibits the activation of TMEM16a by Ca^{2+} [700]. However, elevated Ca-dependent Cl⁻ secretion is not seen in all airways in CF. As shown in Figure 20A, in cultures of human tracheal epithelium, the Ca^{2+}-dependent increase in apical membrane Cl currents is unaltered [354]. Further, in human bronchioles, Ca-dependent Cl⁻ secretion is *reduced* in CF [34].

CFTR increases volume-activated Cl conductances [701], and activates SCL26A9, a Cl⁻ channel that accounts for some of the baseline Cl⁻ secretion in airway epithelia [365]. Wild-type CFTR alters the activity and regulation of a number of K^+ channels [702], activates aquaporin 3 in airway epithelial cells [703], and confers cAMP-dependence on gap junctional channels [704]. CFTR also interacts with carriers: It inhibits Na^+/H^+ exchange [705], and activates apical membrane HCO_3^-/Cl^- exchangers [706], a function probably more important in the pancreas and salivary glands than the airways.

How does CFTR interact with all these various transporters? Evidence obtained with planar lipid bilayers suggests that CFTR can influence the activity of ORDIC by direct physical interaction [707]. However, most of the interactions probably involve PDZ-binding domains on the C-terminal of CFTR [708]. These bind to PDZ motifs on a number of scaffolding proteins that ultimately through various protein–protein interactions link CFTR to other membrane proteins and to the cytoskeleton [709]. A number of regulatory proteins are known to be physically linked to CFTR in this way including the β-adrenergic receptor, adenylate cyclase, protein kinase A, LPA2 (the receptor for the bacterial product lysophosphatidic acid), and MRP4 (that extrudes cAMP) [709]. The PDZ-binding domain of CFTR consists of its final four amino acids (residues 1477–1480). It is noteworthy that a premature stop codon at position 1455 results in loss of the PDZ-binding domain, and causes elevated sweat chloride concentrations but no pancreatic or pulmonary pathology [710].

Many of these interactions have only been detected in expression systems such as Xenopus oocytes, and their relevance to the function of native airway epithelium is unclear. Even in airway epithelium, patch-clamp studies are of necessity done on single cells; the apical membrane of intact cell sheets is too complex to permit patching. And the types of channel expressed in these single, non-polarized cells are often different from those in the apical membrane of intact epithelia [354]. The ORDIC channel in particular may have no real physiological role in intact polarized cell sheets. Further, it is hard to see how CFTR could directly influence more than a small fraction of the population of any given carrier. Carriers in general have turnover rates about a thousand-fold less than channels, and are therefore usually found at much higher densities in cell membranes than channels.

4.4.10 Increased Activation of NFκ-B and Release of Inflammatory Cytokines

There have been multiple reports that airway epithelium is "hyperinflammatory" in CF [553], by which is generally meant that CF cells show constitutive activation of NFκ-B and produce abnormally high amounts of inflammatory cytokines either under baseline conditions or following provocation by bacteria or other inflammatory stimuli. In one particularly dramatic example of this, pieces of human fetal trachea were implanted in SCID mice. The CF grafts had an intraluminal IL-8 content ten times that of non-CF grafts, and significantly more leukocytes in the submucosa [711].

Machen [553] discusses a number of mechanisms which could cause hyperinflammation in CF. These include 1) loss of CFTR input to intracellular signaling pathways, 2) the effects of increased active Na^+ absorption on cell energy supplies, 3) increased acidity of, and lower GSH levels in, ASL, 4) increased Ca^{2+} signaling resulting from ER stress caused by trafficking mutants of CFTR, 5) increased Ca^{2+} influx resulting from hyperpolarization of the basolateral membrane. The possibility that hyperinflammation is triggered by altered pH in intracellular organelles is no longer deemed plausible.

IB-3 cells, a CF airway epithelial cell line, show no mRNA for, or release of, RANTES (Regulated on Activation of Normal T-cell Expressed and presumably Secreted). However, mRNA and release can be induced by transfection with wild-type CFTR, but only if CFTR's PDZ-binding domain is intact. Use of dominant-negative forms of the PDZ-binding protein EBP50 suggested that EBP50 was involved in this CFTR-dependent RANTES expression [712]. These results indicate that CFTR is a member of a macromolecular signaling complex in the plasma membrane that ultimately modulates gene expression in airway epithelial cells. The exact signaling pathways have not been elucidated, however.

AMP-activated kinase influences many aspects of cellular energy homeostasis [713], and the catalytic α subunit of AMP-activated kinase (AMPK) binds to the C-terminal end of CFTR [714] and alters its channel activity [715]. Conversely, AMPK is upregulated by dysfunctional CFTR [716] but this results in *decreased* output of inflammatory cytokines [717]. Direct interactions between CFTR and protein kinase C2 have also been reported, and are disrupted in the ΔF508 mutant [718].

As argued by Machen [553], it seems in general unlikely that CFTR will much influence signaling pathways by protein–protein interactions. This is because CFTR is a very scarce protein. When fully activated, the apical membrane Cl^- conductance in airway epithelium is 4 mS/cm^2 [335]. The unitary conductance of CFTR is ~10 pS [719]. The average apical membrane diameter of airway epithelial cells is ~5 μm. These numbers translate to ~50 copies of CFTR in the membrane. Thus, direct interactions with apical membrane CFTR are likely to comprise an insignificant fraction of the various regulatory inputs on most intracellular signaling pathways.

There is evidence that airway epithelium is relatively hypoxic in CF. Mucosal surfaces of cultures of CF and non-CF airway epithelia were layered with saline to a depth of ~800 μm. At the cell surface, P_{O2} in CF cultures was ~20 mm Hg vs. 50 mm Hg in non-CF cells [720]. It was suggested that the lower P_{O2} in CF was due to enhanced active Na^+ absorption in the CF cells [720]. This hypoxia could then lead to increased production of reactive oxygen species by mitochondria, which in turn could induce alterations in signaling pathways and gene transcription [721], and lead to a hyperinflammatory state. However, recent studies suggest that active Na^+ absorption is not elevated in CF under open-circuit conditions [470, 665], and the mechanism of this CF-related hypoxia is therefore obscure.

Decreased secretion of glutathione in CF could result in increased levels of oxidation in the ASL, and the resulting oxidative stress could potentially activate NFκ-B [722] or other proinflammatory pathways [723]. Increased ASL acidity, likewise, could affect intracellular signaling pathways. Accumulation of misfolded CFTR in airway epithelium increases the volume of ER and the size of its Ca^{2+} stores [724]. Increased leakage or release of Ca^{2+} from the ER then activates

NFκ-B [724]. Finally, by analogy with results on lymphocytes [725], loss of CFTR's Cl⁻ conductance could result in hyperpolarization of the basolateral membrane and increased Ca^{2+} entry via calcium release-activated Ca^{2+} channels (CRAC), again activating NFκ-B [553].

Much of the evidence for a hyperinflammatory state in CF is based on studies with immortalized human airway epithelial cell lines. There are a great many of these from both surface and gland epithelium [210, 726]. Many of them do not form tight junctions and polarize, and they show great variation in cytokine release perhaps in part reflecting the diversity of approaches used in generating them [210]. For instance in one study baseline IL-8 release from a normal cell line was 0.35 ng/µg protein. For two CF lines, it was 0.50 and 0.03 ng/µg protein, respectively. Following stimulation with TNF-α, the corresponding values for the three cell lines were 13.2, 1.3 and 1.9 ng/µg protein [727]. The CF lines were hypoinflammatory! To control for this variation, "matched" pairs of lines have been developed, in which a line derived from a patient with CF is stably transfected (corrected or rescued) with wild-type CFTR. However, the genotype of the founder cell lines is often highly variable, and the corrected cell lines are generally clonally selected. Thus, differences in cytokine release may reflect more the cell of origin than the presence or absence of wild-type CFTR. Overexpression of CFTR may also create problems in the "rescued" cells. For instance, saturation of trafficking pathways may result in delivery of CFTR to the basolateral as well as the apical membrane [728]. Further, if trafficking pathways are overwhelmed with CFTR, trafficking of other proteins will be affected. To control for the effects of overexpression, it is usual to transfect control cells with an irrelevant reporter gene such as lacZ. However, this is not an entirely adequate control as the reporter gene is usually not an integral membrane protein and uses trafficking pathways not used by CFTR. Matched cell lines have also been produced by reducing CFTR function in non-CF cell lines. The 9HTEo- cell line has been stably transfected with plasmids that overproduce the R-domain of CFTR [729]. The R-domain in these so-called pCEP-R cells then blocks the CFTR pore and eliminates cAMP-dependent Cl⁻ secretion. Calu-3 cells are popular for several reasons. First, they form tight junctions and polarize [730]. Second, they contain high levels of CFTR [731]. To eliminate CFTR function Calu-3 cells were stably transfected with CFTR-specific shRNA [732]. The appeal of this approach is that it does not involve expression of exogenous protein.

Work by Aldallal et al. [733] nicely illustrates that even the use of these matched cell lines is problematic; in terms of IL-8 release, different paired cell lines behave differently. The CFTR-complemented cell line, C38, released less IL-8 under baseline conditions and in response to five different inflammatory stimuli than did its parent cell line, IB3, or sham-complemented control cells (Figure 37A). By contrast, CFDo- cells and the rescued CFDE/6REP-CFTR cells produced the same amounts of IL-8 under baseline and in response to four of the same mediators (Figure 37B).

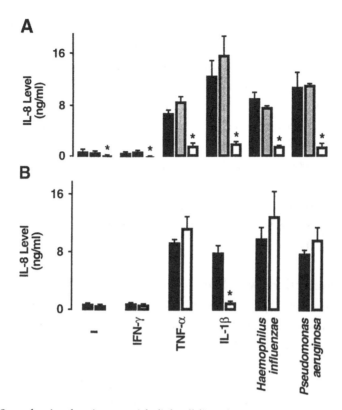

FIGURE 37: IL-8 production by airway epithelial cell lines in response to various inflammatory mediators. A) Black—IB3 cells (a CF cell line); gray—N6 cells, derived from sham-complemented IB3 cells; white—C38 cells, derived by integrated complementation of IB3 cells with wild-type CFTR. B) Black—CFDEo– cells, a CF cell line; white—CFDE/6REP-CFTR cells, episomally complemented with wild-type CFTR. Taken from ref. [733].

Use of transiently transfected cell lines may often be a safer approach. Several different vectors can transfect >50% of the cells in polarized sheets of epithelium without loss of integrity or transport function (the cells maintain their R_{te} and V_{te}). Further, the success of CFTR transfection can be readily determined from the levels of cAMP-dependent I_{sc} in Ussing chambers. The CF15 cell line is derived from the nasal epithelium of a patient homozygous for ΔF508-CFTR. It forms tight junctions and polarizes, developing appreciable R_{te} and I_{sc} [734]. Pizurki et al. [642] used adenovirus for transient transfection of CF15 cells with wild-type CFTR. At least 50% of the cells were transfected, and cAMP-dependent I_{sc} appeared. No changes, however, were seen in the release of IL-8.

Even results obtained with well-differentiated primary cultures should be viewed with caution; there is evidence that the effects of inflammation in the native tissue may persist in primary culture for weeks. Thus, Ribeiro et al. [608] found that primary cultures of ΔF508-CFTR bronchial epithelia at 6–11 days after plating showed enhanced IL-8 release both at baseline and following treatment with bradykinin. By 30–40 days, there was no difference in IL-8 release from CF and non-CF cells. However, treatment of normal cells with supernatant from mucopurulent material caused IL-8 secretion to increase to the same levels as seen in 6- to 11-day-old CF cultures. They concluded that CF-related increases in IL-8 release were mediated by inflammation-induced expansion of the ER and enhanced Ca^{2+} signaling.

Several recent studies on well-differentiated primary cell cultures show little or no CF-induced changes in output of inflammatory cytokines in response to a variety of stimuli [735–737]. Similarly, prolonged treatment of non-CF primary cultures of human tracheal epithelium with a specific blocker of CFTR had little effect on IL-8 release in response to Pseudomonas or a combination of TNF-α plus IL-1β [738].

4.4.11 Altered Interactions with Pseudomonas

Pseudomonas were metabolically labeled with $^{35}SO_4$, and added to primary cultures of nasal polyp cells. Uptake was doubled in CF [739]. However, whereas there were 1.3×10^5 CF cells per well, there were 2.2×10^5 non-CF cells. Clearly there were major differences in the overall morphology of the CF and non-CF cell sheets. In a follow-up study, it was concluded that primary cultures had more asialo-GM1 residues in CF, and that this was a receptor for *Pseudomonas* pilin, one of the major proteins involved in binding of Pseudomonas to cells [740]. Similar results were obtained with CF pulmonary and pancreatic cell lines and their CFTR-rescued pairs, and with the 9HTEo- and pCEP-9 pairing: lack of wild-type CFTR or CFTR function led to increased levels of both asialo-GMs and Pseudomonas binding [741, 742].

Others have been unable to confirm increased binding of Pseudomonas in CF. Hybiske et al. [743], for instance, transfected CF15 cells (homozygous for ΔF508-CFTR) with wild-type CFTR. One or other of two forms of *Pseudomonas aeruginosa* that had been labeled with green fluorescent protein (PAK-GFP and PAO1-GFP) were then added to the mucosal surface. There were no significant differences in PAK or PAO1 binding between the transfected or non-transfected cells. Similarly, another group found that in a variety of polarized cell lines binding of Pseudomonas from the mucosal medium was unaffected by the presence or absence of wild-type CFTR (Figure 38).

Recent studies from several groups suggest that asialo-GM1, though it may bind some laboratory strains of Pseudomonas, is not a major receptor for clinical isolates of this bacterium [745, 746]. Instead, the main receptors may by M-glycan chains on the apical membrane, and heparin sulfate proteoglycans on the basolateral [747]. Further, binding is predominantly to the basolateral membrane [748–750], and therefore in vivo is restricted to areas of epithelial damage.

Whereas some have argued for increased binding of Pseudomonas in CF, others have suggested that CFTR is a receptor for Pseudomonas, and that reduced binding of Pseudomonas by airway epithelium is responsible for the colonization of CF airways with this bacterium! The CFT1 airway epithelial cell line (derived from a ΔF508 homozygote) was stably transfected with wild-type CFTR, a third copy of ΔF508-CFTR or with LacZ. Cells were grown in multi-wells and Pseudomonas added. The cells transfected with wild-type CFTR internalized several times as many Pseudomonas as the parent cell line or the two other transfected lines [751]. Consistent with CFTR being a receptor for Pseudomonas, purified CFTR inhibited internalization of Pseudomonas by human cell lines in vitro, and a synthetic peptide of the first extracellular domain of CFTR inhibited internalization in mice in vivo [752]. Further experiments suggested that binding of bacteria to CFTR results in rapid formation of CFTR-enriched lipid rafts. The bacteria are then taken up by endocytosis, which results in apoptosis, cell sloughing, and clearance of the organisms within the infected cell. In addition, before sloughing, NFκ-B is activated resulting in release of IL-8 and other cytokines. The resulting influx of neutrophils takes care of any Pseudomonas not removed by epithelial sloughing. In the absence of CFTR, bacteria are not internalized and the influx of neutrophils is delayed. The bacteria therefore have more time to proliferate and establish infection [753].

This scheme can be criticized on several grounds. First, the association between bacteria and desquamating cells was based on microscopical data, and it is difficult to determine which comes

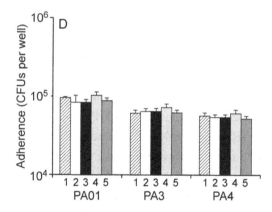

FIGURE 38: Binding of Pseudomonas is unaltered by mutant CFTR. Six hours after adding one or other of 3 different strains of Pseudomonas to the apical surface, the numbers of bacteria associated with the cells was similar in CF and non-CF cell lines. Lines with wild-type CFTR are 16HBE14o- (1) and CFBE14o- clones transfected with wild-type CFTR (4 and 5). Lines with mutant CFTR are CFBE14o- (2) and CFBE14o- control transfected (3). Taken from ref. [744].

first, the binding or the desquamation; bacteria bind preferentially to damaged cells [748]. Second, the studies were done on airway cell lines or on mice in vivo. The mouse has virtually no goblet cells or submucosal glands in its airways [26, 42], and so no mucous blanket, as is also probably true of the cell lines. In human airways in vivo, a mucus barrier is likely to prevent direct interaction of bacteria with the epithelium. Third, flagellin alone activates NFκ-B in epithelial cells [754]. There is thus no need for bacterial uptake to initiate an immune response. Fourth, CFTR is found on the apical membrane between the cilia, and the cilia (and their glycocalyx) would therefore hinder docking of ligand to receptor [68]. Fifth, in airway epithelium, there are ~4 CFTR molecules per μm^2 of apical membrane (see p. 105), and it is hard to see how such a scarce receptor could bind and immobilize a motile Pseudomonas.

Other research has not supported the idea that CFTR is important in Pseudomonas internalization. When CF and rescued cell lines (all with detectable R_{te}) were compared, the rescued lines showed the least internalization [744] (for a list of the cell lines used see legend to Figure 38). Similarly, in polarized airway epithelial cell sheets CFTR was demonstrated to be localized preferentially to the apical membrane, but following exposure to Pseudomonas no intracellular bacteria could be detected. By contrast, non-polarized sheets of the same cell types lacked CFTR in their membranes but internalized Pseudomonas [749]. Recently, others have presented data that internalization of Pseudomonas by mouse tracheal epithelium instead of playing a role in the elimination of the bacteria promotes their eventual development into an antibiotic resistant biofilm [755].

4.4.12 Some Developmental Defects

Submucosal glands extend more distally in the trachea in CF mice than in wild-type mice of the same strain [497]. In the CF pig at birth, tracheal glands are about 50% smaller than normal even though the piglets are not stunted [756].

Nerves containing calcitonin gene-related peptide (CGRP) are found near submucosal glands, and CGRP stimulates gland secretion by a cAMP-dependent mechanism that is abolished in CF. In CF, the levels of CGRP (apparently in the gland epithelial cells) are elevated (presumably as a compensatory response to the inability of this agent to stimulate gland secretion). CGRP is a potent mitogen, and the sustained mitogenic signal in CF somehow leads to loss of stem cells from the submucosal gland cell niche and an increase in stem cells in the surface airway epithelium [401]. Clearly, this redistribution of stem cells will affect repair mechanisms in the CF airway.

4.4.13 Other Changes in CF

Absence of wild-type CFTR hinders epithelial wound healing. In CFTR-deficient Calu-3 cells, cells grew back into denuded areas considerably more slowly than their matched controls [757]. Furthermore, primary cultures of human tracheal epithelium showed a rate of wound healing similar to that of CFTR-replete Calu-3 cells, and in both Calu-3 cells and primary cultures specific pharmacological blockers of CFTR slowed wound healing to a similar extent [757]. Similar results have been obtained by others [758, 759].

Primary cultures of CF human tracheal glands secrete secretory leukocyte protease inhibitor, lactoferrin and lysozyme at rates 10 to 50 times those of non-CF cells. Further, secretory responses to adrenergic and cholinergic agents are reduced in CF [760]. Also in gland cultures, CF is associated with enhanced activity of lysosomal enzymes, an aberration corrected by adenovirus-mediated transfection with wild-type CFTR [761].

In a CF gland cell line (KM4), the ion content of secretory granules was significantly higher and the water content significantly lower than in a non-CF gland cell line (MM-39). Further, secretory granule expansion was deficient in CF. Transfection of CF cells with wild-type CFTR corrected the problems. Conversely, treatment with a specific CFTR inhibitor caused the granules of non-CF cells to resemble those of CF [762].

Altering the amount of CFTR in the apical membrane is one of the ways of regulating Cl secretion [763]. CFTR interacts with trafficking proteins that regulate membrane recycling by endocytosis, and disease-causing mutations that influence endo- and exocytosis of CFTR in airway epithelia have been identified [764].

In immortalized CF tracheal cell lines, cAMP-dependent secretion of glycoconjugates is defective, but can be corrected by transfection with wild-type CFTR [765]. However, it should be noted that in explant cultures of human airway epithelium, goblet cell degranulation is unaltered in CF [71].

Rescue of CFBE41o- cells results in an increase in paracellular electrical resistance in airway cell lines [766]. Inducible nitric oxide synthase (iNOS) is down-regulated in CF [767] due to diminished STAT1 activity [768], and this results in increased susceptibility of airway epithelium to viral infection in CF [769]. Reduced smad3 protein expression in CF leads to impaired TGF-β1 signaling, potentially contributing to the hyperinflammatory state [770]. Apoptosis is compromised in CF, and this may hinder the disposal of bacteria taken up by the airway epithelial cells [771].

4.4.14 Concluding Remarks on Airway Epithelium in CF

Some of the defects in epithelial function reported in CF are expected to have only minor effects on airway pathology. Others have been described only for cell culture systems, and their relevance to native epithelium is questionable. The hyperinflammation hypothesis has not been generally accepted. The idea that enhanced Na^+ absorption inhibits mucociliary clearance by depleting ASL volume is also controversial. No consensus has been reached on whether the binding of Pseudomonas and other bacteria to airway epithelium is altered, or what the result would be if it were. It is clear, however, that gland secretion is altered in CF, and this could contribute to pathology in several ways, such as by increasing mucus viscosity and reducing levels of antimicrobials in ASL. But, CFTR conducts HCO_3^-, and in consequence ASL is abnormally acidic in CF. These changes in HCO_3^- concentration and pH of ASL could have profound effects on a variety of properties of ASL such as mucus viscosity and antimicrobial activity.

·   ·   ·   ·

References

[1]   Wanner A, Salathé M, and O'Riordan TG. Mucociliary clearance in the airways. *Am J Respir Crit Care Med* 154: pp. 1868–902, 1996.

[2]   Lucas AM, and Douglas LC. Principles underlying ciliary activity in the respiratory tract. II. A comparison of nasal clearance in man, monkey and other mammals. *Arch Otolaryngol* 20: pp. 518–41, 1934.

[3]   Sanderson MJ, and Sleigh MA. Ciliary activity of cultured rabbit tracheal epithelium: beat pattern and metachrony. *J Cell Sci* 47: pp. 331–47, 1981.

[4]   Yoneda K. Mucous blanket of rat bronchus: ultrastructural study. *Am Rev Respir Dis* 114: pp. 837–42, 1976.

[5]   Henry BT, Adler J, Hibberd S, Cheema MS, Davis SS, and Rogers TG. Epi-fluorescence microscopy and image analysis used to measure diffusion coefficients in gel systems. *J Pharmacy Pharmacol* 44: pp. 543–9, 1992.

[6]   Hattrup CL, and Gendler SJ. Structure and function of the cell surface (tethered) mucins. *Ann Rev Physiol* 70: pp. 431–57, 2008.

[7]   Widdicombe JH, and Widdicombe JG. Regulation of human airway surface liquid. *Respir Physiol* 99: pp. 3–12, 1995.

[8]   Churg A. Particle uptake by epithelial cells. In: *Particle-Lung Interactions*, edited by Gehr P and Heyder J. New York: Marcel Dekker, Inc., 2000, pp. 401–35.

[9]   Kreyling WG, and Scheuch G. Clearance of particles deposited in the lungs. In: *Particle-Lung Interactions*, edited by Gehr P and Heyder J. New York: Marcel Dekker, Inc., 2000, pp. 323–76.

[10]   Wiedensohler A, Stratmann F, and Tegen I. Environmental particles. In: *Particle-Lung Interactions*, edited by Gehr P and Heyder J. New York: Marcel Dekker, Inc., 2000, pp. 67–88.

[11]   Mauderly JL, Cheng YS, Johnson NF, Hoover MD, and Yeh H-C. Particles inhaled in the occupational setting. In: *Particle-Lung Interactions*, edited by Gehr P and Heyder J. New York: Marcel Dekker, Inc., 2000, pp. 89–170.

[12]   Balashazy I, Horvath A, Sarkany Z, Farkas A, and Hofmann W. Simulation and minimisation of the airway deposition of airborne bacteria. *Inhal Toxicol* 21: pp. 1021–9, 2009.

[13] Schulz H, Brand P, and Heyder J. Particle deposition in the respiratory tract. In: *Particle-Lung Interactions*. New York: Marcel Dekker, Inc., 2000, pp. 229–90.

[14] Heyder J, Gebhart J, Rudolf G, Schiller CF, and Stahlhofen W. Deposition of particles in the human respiratory tract in the size range 0.005-15 µm. *J Aerosol Sci* 17: pp. 811–25, 1986.

[15] Weibel ER. *Morphometry of the Human Lung*. Heidelberg: Springer-Verlag, 1963.

[16] Gerrity TR, Lee PS, Hass FJ, Marinelli A, Werner P, and Lourenco RV. Calculated deposition of inhaled particles in the airway generations of normal subjects. *J Appl Physiol* 47: pp. 867–73, 1979.

[17] Widdicombe JH. The volume of airway surface liquid in health and disease. *Am J Resp Crit Care Med* 165: p. 1566, 2002.

[18] Davis CW, and Dickey BF. Regulated airway goblet cell mucin secretion. *Ann Rev Physiol* 70: pp. 487–512, 2008.

[19] Tos M. Distribution of mucus producing elements in the respiratory tract. Differences between upper and lower airway. *Eur J Respir Dis* 64 Suppl 128: pp. 269–79, 1983.

[20] Broman I. Uber die Entwickelung der konstanten Nasenhohldrusen der Nagetiere. *Z Anat EntwGesch* 60: pp. 439–586, 1921.

[21] Whimster WF. Number and mean volume of individual submucous glands in the human tracheobronchial tree. *Appl Pathol* 4: pp. 24–32, 1986.

[22] Schlesinger RB, and Lippmann M. Particle deposition in casts of the human upper tracheobronchial tree. *Am Ind Hyg Assoc J* 33: pp. 237–51, 1972.

[23] Harkema JR, Mariassy A, St. Geroge J, Hyde DM, and Plopper CG. Epithelial cells of the conducting airways: a species comparison. In: *The Airway Epithelium: Physiology, Pathology, and Pharmacology*, edited by Farmer SG and Hay DWP. New York: Marcel Dekker, Inc., 1991, pp. 3–39.

[24] Thornton DJ, Rousseau K, and McGuckin MA. Structure and function of the polymeric mucins in airways mucus. *Ann Rev Physiol* 70: pp. 459–86, 2008.

[25] Pack RJ, Al-Ugaily LH, and Morris G. The cells of the tracheobronchial epithelium of the mouse: a quantitative light and electron microscopic study. *J Anat* 132: pp. 71–84, 1981.

[26] Widdicombe JH, Chen LL-K, Sporer H, Choi HK, Pecson IS, and Bastacky SJ. Distribution of tracheal and laryngeal mucous glands in some rodents and the rabbit. *J Anat* 198: pp. 207–21, 2001.

[27] Jeffery PK, and Reid L. New observations of rat airway epithelium: a quantitative light and electron microscopic study. *J Anat* 120: pp. 295–320, 1975.

[28] Choi HK, Finkbeiner WE, and Widdicombe JH. A comparative study of mammalian tracheal mucous glands. *J Anat* 197: pp. 361–72, 2000.

[29]   Tos M. Development of the tracheal glands in man. *Acta Pathol Microbiol Scand* Suppl 185: pp. 1–130, 1966.

[30]   Ueki I, German VF, and Nadel J. Micropipette measurement of airway submucosal gland secretion: autonomic effects. *Am Rev Respir Dis* 121: pp. 351–7, 1980.

[31]   Wu DX, Lee CY, Uyekubo SN, Choi HK, Bastacky SJ, and Widdicombe JH. Regulation of the depth of surface liquid in bovine trachea. *Am J Physiol* 274: pp. L388–95, 1998.

[32]   Jiang C, Finkbeiner WE, Widdicombe JH, McCray PB, Jr., and Miller SS. Altered fluid transport across airway epithelium in cystic fibrosis. *Science* 262: pp. 424–7, 1993.

[33]   Knowles MR, Murray GF, Shallal JA, Askin F, Ranga V, Gatzy JT, and Boucher RC. Bioelectric properties and ion flow across excised human bronchi. *J Appl Physiol* 56: pp. 868–77, 1984.

[34]   Blouquit-Laye S, and Chinet T. Ion and liquid transport across the bronchiolar epithelium. *Respir Physiol Neurobiol* 159: pp. 278–82, 2007.

[35]   Shamsuddin AK, and Quinton PM. Surface fluid absorption and secretion in small airways. *J Physiol* 590: pp. 3561–74, 2012.

[36]   Hukkanen J, Pelkonen O, Hakkola J, and Raunio H. Expression and regulation of xenobiotic-metabolizing cytochrome P450 (CYP) enzymes in human lung. *Crit Rev Toxicol* 32: pp. 391–411, 2002.

[37]   Boers JE, Ambergen AW, and Thunnissen FB. Number and proliferation of basal and parabasal cells in normal human airway epithelium. *Am J Respir Crit Care Med* 157: pp. 2000–6, 1998.

[38]   Boers JE, Ambergen AW, and Thunnissen FB. Number and proliferation of Clara cells in normal human airway epithelium. *Am J Respir Crit Care Med* 159: pp. 1585–91, 1999.

[39]   Mercer RR, Russell ML, Roggli VL, and Crapo JD. Cell number and distribution in human and rat airways. *Am J Respir Cell Mol Biol* 10: pp. 613–24, 1994.

[40]   Smith DJ, Gaffney EA, and Blake JR. Modelling mucociliary clearance. *Respir Physiol Neurobiol* 163: pp. 178–88, 2008.

[41]   Matsui H, Randell SH, Perretti SW, Davis CW, and Boucher RC. Coordinated clearance of periciliary liquid and mucus from airway surfaces. *J Clin Invest* 102: pp. 1125–31, 1998.

[42]   Pack RJ, Al-Ugaily LH, Morris G, and Widdicombe JG. The distribution and structure of cells in the tracheal epithelium of the mouse. *Cell Tissue Res* 208: pp. 65–84, 1980.

[43]   Wheeldon EB, Pirie HM, and Breeze RG. A histochemical study of the tracheobronchial epithelial mucosubstances in normal dogs and dogs with chronic bronchitis. *Folia Vet Lat* 6: pp. 45–58, 1976.

[44] Haldiman JT, Henk WG, Henry RW, Albert TF, Abdelbaki YZ, and Duffield DW. Microanatomy of the major airway mucosa of the bowhead whale, *Balaena mysticetus*. *Anat Rec* 209: pp. 219–30, 1984.

[45] Plopper CG, Mariassy AT, Wilson DW, Alley JL, Nishio SJ, and Nettesheim P. Comparison of nonciliated tracheal epithelial cells in six mammalian species: ultrastructure and population densities. *Exp Lung Res* 5: pp. 281–94, 1983.

[46] Yang B, Yu S, Cui Y, He J, Jin X, and Wang R. Histochemical and ultrastructural observations of respiratory epithelium and gland in yak (Bos grunniens). *Anat Rec (Hoboken)* 293: pp. 1259–69, 2010.

[47] Raji AR, and Naserpour M. Light and electron microscopic studies of the trachea in the one-humped camel (Camelus dromedarius). *Anat Histol Embryol* 36: pp. 10–3, 2007.

[48] Jones R, Baskerville A, and Reid L. Histochemical identification of glycoproteins in pig bronchial epithelium: (a) normal and (b) hypertrophied from enzootic pneumonia. *J Pathol* 116: pp. 1–11, 1975.

[49] Gallagher JT, Kent PW, Passatore M, Phipps RJ, and Richardson PS. The composition of tracheal mucus and the nervous control of its secretion in the cat. *Proc Roy Soc Lond B* 192: pp. 49–76, 1975.

[50] Mariassy AT, St. George JA, Nishio SJ, and Plopper CG. Tracheobronchial epithelium of the sheep: III. Carbohydrate histochemical and cytochemical characterization of secretory epithelial cells. *Anat Rec* 22: pp. 540–9, 1988.

[51] Kahwa CKB, and Purton M. Histological and histochemical study of epithelial lining of the respiratory tract in adult goats. *Small Ruminant Research* 20: pp. 181–6, 1996.

[52] Robinson NP, Venning L, and Kyle H. Quantitation of the secretory cells of the ferret tracheobronchial tree. *J Anat* 145: pp. 173–88, 1986.

[53] Li Y, Wang J, He HY, Ma LJ, Zeng J, Deng GC, Liu X, Engelhardt JF, and Wang Y. Immunohistochemical demonstration of airway epithelial cell markers of guinea pig. *Tissue Cell* 43: pp. 283–90, 2011.

[54] Johnson RA, Stauber Z, Hilfer SR, and Kelsen SG. Organization of tracheal epithelium in the cartilaginous portion of adult rabbit and its persistence in organ culture. *Anat Rec* 238: pp. 463–72, 1994.

[55] Christensen G, Breuer R, Hornstra LJ, Lucey C, and Snider GL. The ultrastructure of hamster bronchial epithelium. *Exp Lung Res* 13: pp. 253–77, 1987.

[56] Mair TS, Batten EH, Stokes CR, and Bourne FJ. The histological features of the immune system of the equine respiratory tract. *J Comp Pathol* 97: pp. 575–86, 1987.

[57] Widdicombe JH, and Pecson IS. Distribution and numbers of mucous glands in the horse trachea. *Eq Vet Res* 34: pp. 630–3, 2002.

[58] Widdicombe JH, Basbaum CB, and Highland E. Ion contents and other properties of iso-lated cells from dog tracheal epithelium. *Am J Physiol* 241: pp. C184–92, 1981.

[59] Evans MJ, and Moller PC. Biology of airway basal cells. *Exp Lung Res* 17: pp. 513–31, 1991.

[60] Evans MJ, Van Winkle LS, Fanucchi MV, and Plopper CG. Cellular and molecular char-acteristics of basal cells in airway epithelium. *Exp Lung Res* 27: pp. 401–15, 2001.

[61] Evans MJ, and Plopper CG. The role of basal cells in adhesion of columnar epithelium to airway basement membrane. *Am Rev Respir Dis* 138: pp. 481–2, 1988.

[62] Kawanami O, Ferrans VJ, and Crystal RG. Anchoring fibrils in the normal canine respira-tory system. *Am Rev Respir Dis* 120: pp. 595–611, 1979.

[63] Shum WW, Da Silva N, McKee M, Brown D, and Breton S. Transepithelial projections from basal cells are luminal sensors in pseudostratified epithelia. *Cell* 135: pp. 1108–17, 2008.

[64] Sleigh M. Ciliary adaptations for the propulsion of mucus. *Biorheology* 27: 527–32, 1990.

[65] Lee RJ, and Foskett JK. cAMP-activated Ca^{2+} signaling is required for CFTR-mediated serous cell fluid secretion in porcine and human airways. *J Clin Invest* 120: pp. 3137–48, 2010.

[66] Kreda SM, Mall M, Mengos A, Rochelle L, Yankaskas J, Riordan JR, and Boucher RC. Characterization of wild-type and deltaF508 cystic fibrosis transmembrane regulator in hu-man respiratory epithelia. *Mol Biol Cell* 16: 2154–67, 2005.

[67] Gaillard D, Hinnrasky J, Coscoy S, Hofman P, Matthay MA, Puchelle E, and Barbry P. Early expression of beta- and gamma-subunits of epithelial sodium channel during human airway development. *Am J Physiol* 278: pp. L177–84, 2000.

[68] Enuka Y, Hanukoglu I, Edelheit O, Vaknine H, and Hanukoglu A. Epithelial sodium channels (ENaC) are uniformly distributed on motile cilia in the oviduct and the respiratory airways. *Histochem Cell Biol* 137: pp. 339–53, 2012.

[69] Shah AS, Ben-Shahar Y, Moninger TO, Kline JN, and Welsh MJ. Motile cilia of human airway epithelia are chemosensory. *Science* 325: pp. 1131–4, 2009.

[70] Kikuchi S, Ninomiya T, Kawamata T, Ogasawara N, Kojima T, Tachi N, and Tatsumi H. The acid-sensing ion channel 2 (ASIC2) of ciliated cells in the developing rat nasal septum. *Arch Histol Cytol* 73: pp. 81–9, 2010.

[71] Lethem MI, Dowell ML, Van Scott M, Yankaskas JR, Egan T, Boucher RC, and Davis CW. Nucleotide regulation of goblet cells in human airway epithelial explants: normal exo-cytosis in cystic fibrosis. *Am J Respir Cell Mol Biol* 9: pp. 315–22, 1993.

[72] Rose MC, and Voynow JA. Respiratory tract mucin genes and mucin glycoproteins in health and disease. *Physiol Rev* 86: pp. 245–78, 2006.

[73]   Plopper CG, Hyde DM, and Buckpitt AR. Clara cells. In: *The Lung: Scientific Foundations* (2nd ed.), edited by Crystal RG, West JB, Weibel E and Barnes PJ. Phipadelphia: Lippincott-Raven, 1997, pp. 517–34.

[74]   De Water R, Willems LN, Van Muijen GN, Franken C, Fransen JA, Dijkman JH, and Kramps JA. Ultrastructural localization of bronchial antileukoprotease in central and peripheral human airways by a gold-labeling technique using monoclonal antibodies. *Am Rev Respir Dis* 133: pp. 882–90, 1986.

[75]   Hermans C, and Bernard A. Lung epithelium-specific proteins: characteristics and potential applications as markers. *Am J Respir Crit Care Med* 159: pp. 646–78, 1999.

[76]   Stripp BR, Reynolds SD, Boe IM, Lund J, Power JH, Coppens JT, Wong V, Reynolds PR, and Plopper CG. Clara cell secretory protein deficiency alters Clara cell secretory apparatus and the protein composition of airway lining fluid. *Am J Respir Cell Mol Biol* 27: pp. 170–8, 2002.

[77]   Wong AP, Keating A, and Waddell TK. Airway regeneration: the role of the Clara cell secretory protein and the cells that express it. *Cytotherapy* 11: pp. 676–87, 2009.

[78]   Van Scott MR, Davis CW, and Boucher RC. Na^+ and Cl^- transport across rabbit nonciliated bronchiolar epithelial (Clara) cells. *Am J Physiol* 256: pp. C893–901, 1989.

[79]   Van Scott MR, Chinet TC, Burnette AD, and Paradiso AM. Purinergic regulation of ion transport across nonciliated bronchiolar epithelial (Clara) cells. *Am J Physiol* 269: pp. L30–7, 1995.

[80]   Van Scott MR, Penland CM, Welch CA, and Lazarowski E. Beta-adrenergic regulation of Cl^- and HCO_3^- secretion by Clara cells. *Am J Respir Cell Mol Biol* 13: pp. 344–51, 1995.

[81]   Chinet TC, Gabriel SE, Penland CM, Sato M, Stutts MJ, Boucher RC, and Van Scott MR. CFTR-like chloride channels in non-ciliated bronchiolar epithelial (Clara) cells. *Biochem Biophys Res Commun* 230: pp. 470–5, 1997.

[82]   Evans MJ, Cabral-Anderson LJ, and Freeman G. Role of the Clara cell in renewal of the bronchiolar epithelium. *Lab Invest* 38: pp. 648–55, 1978.

[83]   Breuer R, Christensen TG, Wax Y, Bolbochan G, Lucey EC, Stone PJ, and Snider GL. Relationship of secretory granule content and proliferative intensity in the secretory compartment of the hamster bronchial epithelium. *Am J Respir Cell Mol Biol* 8: pp. 480–5, 1993.

[84]   Jeffery PK. Morphologic features of airway surface epithelial cells and glands. *Am Rev Respir Dis* 128: pp. S14–20, 1983.

[85]   Rogers AV, Dewar A, Corrin B, and Jeffery PK. Identification of serous-like cells in the surface epithelium of human bronchioles. *Eur Respir J* 6: pp. 498–504, 1993.

[86]   Huang HT, Haskell A, and McDonald DM. Changes in epithelial secretory cells and potentiation of neurogenic inflammation in the trachea of rats with respiratory tract infections. *Anat Embryol (Berl)* 180: pp. 325–41, 1989.

[87]   Randell SH. Airway epithelial stem cells and the pathophysiology of chronic obstructive pulmonary disease. *Proc Am Thorac Soc* 3: pp. 718–25, 2006.

[88]   Sorokin SP, and Hoyt RF. Neuropepithelial bodies and solitary small-granule cells. In: *Lung Cell Biology*, edited by Massaro D. New York: Marcel Dekker, 1989, pp. 191–344.

[89]   Van Lommel A, Bolle T, Fannes W, and Lauweryns JM. The pulmonary neuroendocrine system: the past decade. *Arch Histol Cytol* 62: pp. 1–16, 1999.

[90]   Degan S, Lopez GY, Kevill K, and Sunday ME. Gastrin-releasing peptide, immune responses, and lung disease. *Ann N Y Acad Sci* 1144: pp. 136–47, 2008.

[91]   Sbarbati A, and Osculati F. A new fate for old cells: brush cells and related elements. *J Anat* 206: pp. 349–58, 2005.

[92]   Krasteva G, Canning BJ, Hartmann P, Veres TZ, Papadakis T, Muhlfeld C, Schliecker K, Tallini YN, Braun A, Hackstein H, Baal N, Weihe E, Schutz B, Kotlikoff M, Ibanez-Tallon I, and Kummer W. Cholinergic chemosensory cells in the trachea regulate breathing. *Proc Natl Acad Sci USA* 108: pp. 9478–83, 2011.

[93]   Tizzano M, Gulbransen BD, Vandenbeuch A, Clapp TR, Herman JP, Sibhatu HM, Churchill ME, Silver WL, Kinnamon SC, and Finger TE. Nasal chemosensory cells use bitter taste signaling to detect irritants and bacterial signals. *Proc Natl Acad Sci USA* 107: pp. 3210–5, 2010.

[94]   Davidson DJ, Gray MA, Kilanowski FM, Tarran R, Randell SH, Sheppard DN, Argent BE, and Dorin JR. Murine epithelial cells: isolation and culture. *J Cyst Fibros* 3 Suppl 2: pp. 59–62, 2004.

[95]   Matsuba K, Takizawa T, and Thurlbeck WM. Oncocytes in human bronchial mucous glands. *Thorax* 24: pp. 181–5, 1972.

[96]   Meyrick B, and Reid L. Ultrastucture of cells in human bronchial submucosal glands. *J Anat* 107: pp. 291–9, 1970.

[97]   Guaraldi F, Zang G, Dackiw AP, and Caturegli P. Oncocytic mania: a review of oncocytic lesions throughout the body. *J Endocrinol Invest* 34: pp. 383–94, 2011.

[98]   Kawamata S, and Fujita H. Fine structural aspects of the development and aging of the tracheal epithelium of mice. *Arch Histol Jpn* 46: pp. 355–72, 1983.

[99]   Pilette C, Durham SR, Vaerman JP, and Sibille Y. Mucosal immunity in asthma and chronic obstructive pulmonary disease: a role for immunoglobulin A? *Proc Am Thorac Soc* 1: pp. 125–35, 2004.

[100] Akpavie SO, and Pirie HM. Globule leukocytes and bovine parasitic bronchitis. *Anat Histol Embryol* 22: pp. 144–50, 1993.

[101] Sertl K, Takemura T, Tschachler E, Ferrans VJ, Kaliner MA, and Shevach EM. Dendritic cells with antigen-presenting capability reside in airway epithelium, lung parenchyma, and visceral pleura. *J Exp Med* 163: pp. 436–51, 1986.

[102] Weichselbaum M, Sparrow MP, Hamilton EJ, Thompson PJ, and Knight DA. A confocal microscopic study of solitary pulmonary neuroendocrine cells in human airway epithelium. *Respir Res* 6: p. 115, 2005.

[103] Wine JJ. Parasympathetic control of airway submucosal glands: central reflexes and the airway intrinsic nervous system. *Auton Neurosci* 133: pp. 35–54, 2007.

[104] Carr MJ, and Undem BJ. Bronchopulmonary afferent nerves. *Respirology* 8: pp. 291–301, 2003.

[105] McDowell EM, Newkirk C, and Coleman B. Development of hamster tracheal epithelium: I. A quantitative morphologic study in the fetus. *Anat Rec* 213: pp. 429–47, 1985.

[106] Plopper CG, Alley JL, and Weir AJ. Differentiation of tracheal epithelium during fetal lung maturation in the rhesus monkey Macaca mulata. *Am J Anat* 175: pp. 59–71, 1986.

[107] McDowell EM, Newkirk C, and Coleman B. Development of hamster tracheal epithelium: II. Cell proliferation in the fetus. *Anat Rec* 213: pp. 448–56, 1985.

[108] Evans MJ, Shami SG, Cabral-Anderson LJ, and Dekker NP. Role of nonciliated cells in renewal of the bronchial epithelium of rats exposed to NO_2. *Am J Pathol* 123: pp. 126–33, 1986.

[109] Otani EM, Newkirk C, and McDowell EM. Development of hamster tracheal epithelium: IV. cell proliferation and cytodifferentiation in the neonate. *Anat Rec* 214: pp. 183–92, 1986.

[110] Leigh MW, Gambling TM, Carson JL, Collier AM, Wood RE, and Boat TF. Postnatal development of tracheal surface epithelium and submucosal glands in the ferret. *Exp Lung Res* 10: pp. 153–69, 1986.

[111] Smolich JJ, Stratford BF, Maloney JE, and Ritchie BC. Postnatal development of the epithelium of larynx and trachea in the rat: Scanning electron microscopy. *J Anat* 124: pp. 657–73, 1976.

[112] Ayers MM, and Jeffery PK. Proliferation and differentiation in mammalian airway epithelium. *Eur Respir J* 1: pp. 58–80, 1988.

[113] Wright N, and Alison M. *The Biology of Epithelial Cell Populations*. Oxford: Clarendon Press, 1984.

[114] Breuer R, Zajicek G, Christensen TG, Lucey EC, and Snider GL. Cell kinetics of normal adult hamster bronchial epithelium in the steady state. *Am J Respir Cell Mol Biol* 2: pp. 51–8, 1990.

[115] Rock JR, Onaitis MW, Rawlins EL, Lu Y, Clark CP, Xue Y, Randell SH, and Hogan BL. Basal cells as stem cells of the mouse trachea and human airway epithelium. *Proc Natl Acad Sci USA* 106: pp. 12771–5, 2009.

[116] Rock JR, and Hogan BLM. Epithelial progenitor cells in lung development, maintenance, repair, and disease. *Ann Rev Cell Dev Biol* 27: pp. 493–512, 2011.

[117] Rawlins EL, Okubo T, Xue Y, Brass DM, Auten RL, Hasegawa H, Wang F, and Hogan BL. The role of Scgb1a1+ Clara cells in the long-term maintenance and repair of lung airway, but not alveolar, epithelium. *Cell Stem Cell* 4: pp. 525–34, 2009.

[118] Hong KU, Reynolds SD, Giangreco A, Hurley CM, and Stripp BR. Clara cell secretory protein-expressing cells of the airway neuroepithelial body microenvironment include a label-retaining subset and are critical for epithelial renewal after progenitor cell depletion. *Am J Respir Cell Mol Biol* 24: pp. 671–81, 2001.

[119] Johnson NF, and Hubbs AF. Epithelial progenitor cells in the rat trachea. *Am J Respir Cell Mol Biol* 3: pp. 579–85, 1990.

[120] Rawlins EL, Ostrowski LE, Randell SH, and Hogan BL. Lung development and repair: contribution of the ciliated lineage. *Proc Natl Acad Sci USA* 104: pp. 410–7, 2007.

[121] Liu X, and Engelhardt JF. The glandular stem/progenitor cell niche in airway development and repair. *Proc Am Thorac Soc* 5: pp. 682–8, 2008.

[122] Voynow JA, and Rubin BK. Mucins, mucus, and sputum. *Chest* 135: pp. 505–12, 2009.

[123] Curran DR, and Cohn L. Advances in mucous cell metaplasia: a plug for mucus as a therapeutic focus in chronic airway disease. *Am J Respir Cell Mol Biol* 42: pp. 268–75, 2010.

[124] Tesfaigzi Y. Roles of apoptosis in airway epithelium. *Am J Respir Cell Mol Biol* 34: pp. 537–47, 2006.

[125] Rock JR, Randell SH, and Hogan BL. Airway basal stem cells: a perspective on their roles in epithelial homeostasis and remodeling. *Dis Model Mech* 3: pp. 545–56, 2010.

[126] Jetten AM. Growth and differentiation factors in tracheobronchial epithelium. *Am J Physiol* 260: pp. L361–73, 1991.

[127] Herfs M, Hubert P, Poirrier AL, Vandevenne P, Renoux V, Habraken Y, Cataldo D, Boniver J, and Delvenne P. Pro-inflammatory cytokines induce bronchial hyperplasia and squamous metaplasia in smokers: implications for COPD therapy. *Am J Respir Cell Mol Biol* 47: pp. 67–79, 2012.

[128] Fromter E, and Diamond J. Route of passive ion permeation in epithelia. *Nature New Biology* 235: pp. 9–13, 1972.

[129] Spring K. Epithelial Fluid Transport—a century of investigation. *News Physiol Sci* 14: pp. 92–8, 1999.

[130] Matsui H, Davis CW, Tarran R, and Boucher RC. Osmotic water permeabilities of cultured, well-differentiated normal and cystic fibrosis airway epithelia. *J Clin Invest* 105: pp. 1419–27, 2000.

[131] Folkesson HG, Matthay MA, Frigeri A, and Verkman AS. Transepithelial water permeability in microperfused distal airways. Evidence for channel-mediated water transport. *J Clin Invest* 97: pp. 664–71, 1996.

[132] Pedersen PS, Procida K, Larsen PL, Holstein-Rathlou NH, and Frederiksen O. Water permeability in human airway epithelium. *Pflugers Arch* 451: pp. 464–73, 2005.

[133] Novotny JA, and Jakobsson E. Computational studies of ion-water flux coupling in the airway epithelium. I. Construction of model. *Am J Physiol* 270: pp. C1751–63, 1996.

[134] Novotny JA, and Jakobsson E. Computational studies of ion-water flux coupling in the airway epithelium. II. Role of specific transport mechanisms. *Am J Physiol* 270: pp. C1764–72, 1996.

[135] Welsh MJ, Widdicombe JH, and Nadel JA. Fluid transport across the canine tracheal epithelium. *J Appl Physiol* 49: pp. 905–9, 1980.

[136] Finkbeiner WE, and Widdicombe JH. Control of nasal airway secretions, ion transport, and water movement. In: *Treatise on Pulmonary Toxicology. Volume 1. Comparative Biology of the Normal Lung*, edited by Parent RA. Boca Raton, FL: CRC Press, 1992, pp. 633–57.

[137] Welsh MJ, and Widdicombe JH. Pathways of ion movement in the canine tracheal epithelium. *Am J Physiol* 239: pp. F215–21, 1980.

[138] Watson CJ, Rowland M, and Warhurst G. Functional modeling of tight junctions in intestinal cell monolayers using polyethylene glycol oligomers. *Am J Physiol* 281: pp. C388–97, 2001.

[139] Man SF, Hulbert WC, Mok K, Ryan T, and Thomson AB. Effects of sulfur dioxide on pore populations of canine tracheal epithelium. *J Appl Physiol* 60: pp. 416–26, 1986.

[140] Mariano C, Sasaki H, Brites D, and Brito MA. A look at tricellulin and its role in tight junction formation and maintenance. *Eur J Cell Biol* 90: pp. 787–96, 2011.

[141] Schneeberger EE. Heterogeneity of tight junction morphology in extrapulmonary and intrapulmonary airways of the rat. *Anat Rec* 198: pp. 193–208, 1980.

[142] Godfrey RW. Human airway epithelial tight junctions. *Microsc Res Tech* 38: pp. 488–99, 1997.

[143] Coyne CB, Vanhook MK, Gambling TM, Carson JL, Boucher RC, and Johnson LG. Regulation of airway tight junctions by proinflammatory cytokines. *Mol Biol Cell* 13: pp. 3218–34, 2002.

[144] Claude P. Morphological factors influencing transepithelial permeabilty: A model for the resistance of the zonula occludens. *J Membrane Biol* 39: pp. 219–32, 1978.

[145] Schneeberger EE, and McCormack JM. Intercellular junctions in upper airway submucosal glands of the rat: a tracer and freeze fracture study. *Anat Rec* 210: pp. 421–33, 1984.

[146] Roesinger B, Schiller A, and Taugner R. A freeze-fracture study of tight junctions in the pars convoluta and pars recta of the renal proximal tubule. *Cell Tissue Res* 186: pp. 121–33, 1978.

[147] Zeuthen T. General models for water transport across leaky epithelia. In: *Molecular Mecha-*

nisms of Water Transport across Biological Membranes, edited by Zeuthen T and Stein WD. San Diego: Academic Press, 2002, pp. 285–316.

[148] Boucher RC, Ranga V, Pare PD, Inoue S, Moroz LA, and Hogg JC. Effect of histamine and methacholine on guinea pig tracheal permeability to HRP. *J Appl Physiol* 45: pp. 939–48, 1978.

[149] Rangachari PK, and McWade D. Peptides increase anion conductance of canine trachea: an effect on tight junctions. *Biochim Biophys Acta* 863: pp. 305–8, 1986.

[150] Poulsen AN, Klausen TL, Pedersen PS, Willumsen NJ, and Frederiksen O. Nucleotide regulation of paracellular Cl⁻ permeability in natural rabbit airway epithelium. *Pflugers Arch* 452: pp. 188–98, 2006.

[151] Unwalla HJ, Horvath G, Roth FD, Conner GE, and Salathe M. Albuterol modulates its own transepithelial flux via changes in paracellular permeability. *Am J Respir Cell Mol Biol* 46: pp. 551–8, 2012.

[152] Flynn AN, Itani OA, Moninger TO, and Welsh MJ. Acute regulation of tight junction ion selectivity in human airway epithelia. *Proc Natl Acad Sci USA* 106: pp. 3591–6, 2009.

[153] van Os CH, Wiedner G, and Wright EM. Volume flows across gallbladder epithelium induced by small hydrostatic and osmotic gradients. *J Memb Biol* 49: pp. 1–20, 1979.

[154] Azizi F, Matsumoto PS, Wu DX, and Widdicombe JH. Effects of hydrostatic pressure on permeability of airway epithelium. *Exp Lung Res* 23: pp. 257–67, 1997.

[155] Kondo M, Finkbeiner WE, and Widdicombe JH. Changes in permeability of dog tracheal epithelium in response to hydrostatic pressure. *Am J Physiol* 262: pp. L176–82, 1992.

[156] Barnes PJ. Neurogenic inflammation in the airways. *Respir Physiol* 125: pp. 145–54, 2001.

[157] Serikov VB, Jang YJ, and Widdicombe JH. An estimate of the subepithelial pressure that drives inflammatory transudate into the airway lumen. *J Appl Physiol* 92: pp. 1702–8, 2002.

[158] Zemans RL, Colgan SP, and Downey GP. Transepithelial migration of neutrophils: mechanisms and implications for acute lung injury. *Am J Respir Cell Mol Biol* 40: pp. 519–35, 2009.

[159] Burns AR, Smith CW, and Walker DC. Unique structural features that influence neutrophil emigration into the lung. *Physiol Rev* 83: pp. 309–36, 2003.

[160] Kondo M, Tamaoki J, Takeyama K, Nakata J, and Nagai A. Interleukin-13 induces goblet cell differentiation in primary cell culture from guinea pig tracheal epithelium. *Am J Respir Cell Mol Biol* 27: pp. 536–41, 2002.

[161] Vermeer PD, Einwalter LA, Moninger TO, Rokhlina T, Kern JA, Zabner J, and Welsh MJ. Segregation of receptor and ligand regulates activation of epithelial growth factor receptor. *Nature* 422: pp. 322–6, 2003.

[162] Lamblin G, Degroote S, Perini JM, Delmotte P, Scharfman A, Davril M, Lo-Guidice JM, Houdret N, Dumur V, Klein A, and Rousse P. Human airway mucin glycosylation:

a combinatory of carbohydrate determinants which vary in cystic fibrosis. *Glycoconj J* 18: pp. 661–84, 2001.

[163] Kim KC. Role of epithelial mucins during airway infection. *Pulm Pharmacol Ther*, 2011 Dec 17. [Epub ahead of print].

[164] Bobek LA, Liu J, Sait SN, Shows TB, Bobek YA, and Levine MJ. Structure and chromosomal localization of the human salivary mucin gene, MUC7. *Genomics* 31: pp. 277–82, 1996.

[165] Sharma P, Dudus L, Nielsen PA, Clausen H, Yankaskas JR, Hollingsworth MA, and Engelhardt JF. MUC5B and MUC7 are differentially expressed in mucous and serous cells of submucosal glands in human bronchial airways. *Am J Respir Cell Mol Biol* 19: pp. 30–7, 1998.

[166] Levine MJ, Reddy MS, Tabak LA, Loomis RE, Bergey EJ, Jones PC, Cohen RE, Stinson MW, and Al-Hashimi I. Structural aspects of salivary glycoproteins. *J Dent Res* 66: pp. 436–41, 1987.

[167] Tabak LA. In defense of the oral cavity: structure, biosynthesis, and function of saliray mucins. *Ann Rev Physiol* 57: pp. 547–64, 1995.

[168] Finkbeiner WE, Zlock LT, Morikawa M, Lao AY, Dasari V, and Widdicombe JH. Cystic fibrosis and the relationship between mucin and chloride secretion by differentiated cultures of human airway gland mucous cells. *Am J Physiol* 301: pp. L402–14, 2011.

[169] Groneberg DA, Eynott PR, Oates T, Lim S, Wu R, Carlstedt I, Nicholson AG, and Chung KF. Expression of MUC5AC and MUC5B mucins in normal and cystic fibrosis lung. *Respir Med* 96: pp. 81–6, 2002.

[170] Caramori G, Casolari P, Di Gregorio C, Saetta M, Baraldo S, Boschetto P, Ito K, Fabbri LM, Barnes PJ, Adcock IM, Cavallesco G, Chung KF, and Papi A. MUC5AC expression is increased in bronchial submucosal glands of stable COPD patients. *Histopathology* 55: pp. 321–31, 2009.

[171] Zhu L, Lee P, Yu D, Tao S, and Chen Y. Cloning and characterization of human MUC19 gene. *Am J Respir Cell Mol Biol* 45: pp. 348–58, 2011.

[172] Martinez-Anton A, Debolos C, Garrido M, Roca-Ferrer J, Barranco C, Alobid I, Xaubet A, Picado C, and Mullol J. Mucin genes have different expression patterns in healthy and diseased upper airway mucosa. *Clin Exp Allergy* 36: pp. 448–57, 2006.

[173] Moon UY, Kim CH, Choi JY, Kim YJ, Choi YH, Yoon HG, Kim H, and Yoon JH. AP2alpha is essential for MUC8 gene expression in human airway epithelial cells. *J Cell Biochem* 110: pp. 1386–98, 2010.

[174] Basbaum C, Lemjabbar H, Longphre M, Li D, Gensch E, and McNamara N. Control of mucin transcription by diverse injury-induced signaling pathways. *Am J Respir Crit Care Med* 160: pp. S44–8, 1999.

[175]   Perez-Vilar J. Mucin granule intraluminal organization. *Am J Respir Cell Mol Biol* 36: pp. 183–90, 2007.

[176]   Verdugo P. Mucin exocytosis. *Am Rev Respir Dis* 144: pp. S33–7, 1991.

[177]   Sheehan JK, Kesimer M, and Pickles R. Innate immunity and mucus structure and function. *Novartis Found Symp* 279: pp. 155–66, 2006.

[178]   Davies JR, Kirkham S, Svitacheva N, Thornton DJ, and Carlstedt I. MUC16 is produced in tracheal surface epithelium and submucosal glands and is present in secretions from normal human airway and cultured bronchial epithelial cells. *Int J Biochem Cell Biol* 39: pp. 1943–54, 2007.

[179]   Theodoropoulos G, Carraway CA, and Carraway KL. MUC4 involvement in ErbB2/ErbB3 phosphorylation and signaling in response to airway cell mechanical injury. *J Cell Biochem* 107: pp. 112–22, 2009.

[180]   Simon GC, Martin RJ, Smith S, Thaikoottathil J, Bowler RP, Barenkamp SJ, and Chu HW. Up-regulation of MUC18 in airway epithelial cells by IL-13: implications in bacterial adherence. *Am J Respir Cell Mol Biol* 44: pp. 606–13, 2011.

[181]   Davis C, Dowell M, Lethem M, and Van Scott M. Goblet cell degranulation in isolated tracheal epithelium: response to exogenous ATP, ADP, and adenosine. *Am J Physiol* 262: pp. C1313–23, 1993.

[182]   Tokuyama K, Kuo HP, Rhode JA, Barnes PJ, and Rogers DF. Neural control of goblet cell secretion in guinea pig airways. *Am J Physiol* 259: pp. L108–15, 1990.

[183]   Kim KC, Nassiri J, and Brody JS. Mechanisms of airway goblet cell mucin release: studies with cultured tracheal surface epithelial cells. *Am J Respir Cell Mol Biol* 1: pp. 137–43, 1989.

[184]   Kim KC, and Brody JS. Use of primary cell culture to study regulation of airway surface epithelial mucus secretion. *Symp Soc Exp Biol* 43: pp. 231–9, 1989.

[185]   Kim KC, Wasano K, Niles RM, Schuster JE, Stone PJ, and Brody JS. Human neutrophil elastase releases cell surface mucins from primary cultures of hamster tracheal epithelial cells. *Proc Natl Acad Sci USA* 84: pp. 9304–8, 1987.

[186]   Sheppard MN, Kurian SS, Henzen-Longmans SC, Michetti F, Cocchia D, Cole P, Rush RA, Marangos PJ, Bloom SR, and Polak JM. Neuron-specific enolase and s-100: new markers for delineating the innervation of the respiratory tract in man and other animals. *Thorax* 38: pp. 333–40, 1983.

[187]   Mak JCW, and Barnes, P.J. Autoradiographic visualization of muscarinic receptor subtypes in human and guinea pig lung. *Am Rev Respir Dis* 141: pp. 1559–68, 1990.

[188]   Mak JC, Grandordy B, and Barnes PJ. High affinity [^{3}H]formoterol binding sites in lung: characterization and autoradiographic mapping. *Eur J Pharmacol* 269: pp. 35–41, 1994.

[189] Kim K, McCracken, K, Lee, BC, Shin, CY, Jo, MJ, Lee, CJ, Ko, KH. Airway goblet cell mucin: its structure and regulation of secretion. *Eur Respir J* 10: pp. 2644–9, 1997.

[190] McDonald DM. Neurogenic inflammation in rat trachea. I. Changes in venules, leukocytes, and epithelial cells. *J Neurocytol* 17: pp. 583–603, 1988.

[191] Grygorczyk R, and Hanrahan JW. CFTR-independent ATP release from epithelial cells triggered by mechanical stimuli. *Am J Physiol* 272: pp. C1058–66, 1997.

[192] Rogers DF. Airway goblet cells: responsive and adaptable front-line defenders. *Eur Respir J* 7: pp. 1690–706, 1994.

[193] Kim KC. Epithelial cell goblet secretion. In: *Airway Secretion*, edited by Takishima T and Shimura S. New York: Marcel Dekker, Inc., 1994, pp. 433–50.

[194] Takeyama K, Agusti C, Ueki I, Lausier J, Cardell LO, and Nadel JA. Neutrophil-dependent goblet cell degranulation: role of membrane-bound elastase and adhesion molecules. *Am J Physiol* 275: pp. L294–302, 1998.

[195] Park JA, He F, Martin LD, Li Y, Chorley BN, and Adler KB. Human neutrophil elastase induces hypersecretion of mucin from well-differentiated human bronchial epithelial cells in vitro via a protein kinase C{delta}-mediated mechanism. *Am J Pathol* 167: pp. 651–61, 2005.

[196] Tamaoki J, Nakata J, Tagaya E, and Konno K. Effects of roxithromycin and erythromycin on interleukin 8-induced neutrophil recruitment and goblet cell secretion in guinea pig tracheas. *Antimicrob Agents Chemother* 40: pp. 1726–8, 1996.

[197] Savoie C, Plant M, Zwikker M, van Staden CJ, Boulet L, Chan CC, Rodger IW, and Pon DJ. Effect of dexamethasone on antigen-induced high molecular weight glycoconjugate secretion in allergic guinea pigs. *Am J Respir Cell Mol Biol* 13: pp. 133–43, 1995.

[198] Kim KC. Biochemistry and pharmacology of mucin-like glycoproteins produced by cultured airway epithelial cells. *Exp Lung Res* 17: pp. 533–45, 1991.

[199] Abdullah LH, Conway JD, Cohn JA, and Davis CW. Protein kinase C and Ca^{2+} activation of mucin secretion in airway goblet cells. *Am J Physiol* 273: pp. L201–10, 1997.

[200] Kesimer M, Scull M, Brighton B, DeMaria G, Burns K, O'Neal W, Pickles RJ, and Sheehan JK. Characterization of exosome-like vesicles released from human tracheobronchial ciliated epithelium: a possible role in innate defense. *FASEB J* 23: pp. 1858–68, 2009.

[201] Vareille M, Kieninger E, Edwards MR, and Regamey N. The airway epithelium: soldier in the fight against respiratory viruses. *Clin Microbiol Rev* 24: pp. 210–29, 2011.

[202] Kolls JK, McCray PB, Jr., and Chan YR. Cytokine-mediated regulation of antimicrobial proteins. *Nat Rev Immunol* 8: pp. 829–35, 2008.

[203] Candiano G, Bruschi M, Pedemonte N, Musante L, Ravazzolo R, Liberatori S, Bini L, Galietta LJ, and Zegarra-Moran O. Proteomic analysis of the airway surface liquid: modulation by proinflammatory cytokines. *Am J Physiol* 292: pp. L185–98, 2007.

[204]   Kesimer M, Kirkham S, Pickles RJ, Henderson AG, Alexis NE, Demaria G, Knight D, Thornton DJ, and Sheehan JK. Tracheobronchial air-liquid interface cell culture: a model for innate mucosal defense of the upper airways? *Am J Physiol* 296: pp. L92–100, 2009.

[205]   Ali M, Lillehoj EP, Park Y, Kyo Y, and Kim KC. Analysis of the proteome of human airway epithelial secretions. *Proteome Sci* 9: 4, 2011.

[206]   Dubin RF, Robinson SK, and Widdicombe JH. Secretion of lactoferrin and lysozyme by cultures of human airway epithelium. *Am J Physiol* 286: pp. L750–5, 2004.

[207]   Bowes D, Clark AE, and Corrin B. Ultrastructural localisation of lactoferrin and glycoprotein in human bronchial glands. *Thorax* 36: pp. 108–15, 1981.

[208]   Bowes D, and Corrin B. Ultrastructural immunocytochemical localisation of lysozyme in human bronchial glands. *Thorax* 32: pp. 163–70, 1977.

[209]   Dvorak A, Tilley AE, Shaykhiev R, Wang R, and Crystal RG. Do airway epithelium air-liquid cultures represent the in vivo airway epithelium transcriptome? *Am J Respir Cell Mol Biol* 44: pp. 465–73, 2011.

[210]   Rochwerger L, and Buchwald M. Cell cultures in cystic fibrosis research. In: *Cystic Fibrosis—Current Topics*, edited by Dodge J, Brock D and Widdicombe J. Chichester: John Wiley & Sons, 1996, pp. 1–37.

[211]   Bals R, Wang X, Wu Z, Freeman T, Bafna V, Zasloff M, and Wilson JM. Human beta-defensin 2 is a salt-sensitive peptide antibiotic expressed in human lung. *J Clin Invest* 102: pp. 874–80, 1998.

[212]   Singh PK, Jia HP, Wiles K, Hesselberth J, Liu L, Conway BA, Greenberg EP, Valore EV, Welsh MJ, Ganz T, Tack BF, and McCray PB. Production of β-defensins by human airway epithelia. *Proc Natl Acad Sci USA* 95: pp. 14961–6, 1998.

[213]   Bals R, Wang X, Zasloff M, and Wilson JM. The peptide antibiotic LL-37/hCAP-18 is expressed in epithelia of the human lung where it has broad antimicrobial activity at the airway surface. *Proc Natl Acad Sci USA* 95: pp. 9541–6, 1998.

[214]   Frazier MD, Mamo LB, Ghio AJ, and Turi JL. Hepcidin expression in human airway epithelial cells is regulated by interferon-gamma. *Respir Res* 12: p. 100, 2011.

[215]   Nicholas BL, Skipp P, Barton S, Singh D, Bagmane D, Mould R, Angco G, Ward J, Guha-Niyogi B, Wilson S, Howarth P, Davies DE, Rennard S, O'Connor CD, and Djukanovic R. Identification of lipocalin and apolipoprotein A1 as biomarkers of chronic obstructive pulmonary disease. *Am J Respir Crit Care Med* 181: pp. 1049–60, 2010.

[216]   Starner TD, Barker CK, Jia HP, Kang Y, and McCray PB, Jr. CCL20 is an inducible product of human airway epithelia with innate immune properties. *Am J Respir Cell Mol Biol* 29: pp. 627–33, 2003.

[217]   Eliasson M, Morgelin M, Farber JM, Egesten A, and Albiger B. Streptococcus pneumoniae induces expression of the antibacterial CXC chemokine MIG/CXCL9 via MyD88-

dependent signaling in a murine model of airway infection. *Microbes Infect* 12: pp. 565–73, 2010.

[218] John G, Chillappagari S, Rubin BK, Gruenert DC, and Henke MO. Reduced surface toll-like receptor-4 expression and absent interferon-gamma-inducible protein-10 induction in cystic fibrosis airway cells. *Exp Lung Res* 37: pp. 319–26, 2011.

[219] Porter JC, Falzon M, and Hall A. Polarized localization of epithelial CXCL11 in chronic obstructive pulmonary disease and mechanisms of T cell egression. *J Immunol* 180: pp. 1866–77, 2008.

[220] Tieu DD, Peters AT, Carter RG, Suh L, Conley DB, Chandra R, Norton J, Grammer LC, Harris KE, Kato A, Kern RC, and Schleimer RP. Evidence for diminished levels of epithelial psoriasin and calprotectin in chronic rhinosinusitis. *J Allergy Clin Immunol* 125: pp. 667–75, 2010.

[221] Bartlett JA, Gakhar L, Penterman J, Singh PK, Mallampalli RK, Porter E, and McCray PB, Jr. PLUNC: a multifunctional surfactant of the airways. *Biochem Soc Trans* 39: pp. 1012–6, 2011.

[222] Bingle CD, Wilson K, Lunn H, Barnes FA, High AS, Wallace WA, Rassl D, Campos MA, Ribeiro M, and Bingle L. Human LPLUNC1 is a secreted product of goblet cells and minor glands of the respiratory and upper aerodigestive tracts. *Histochem Cell Biol* 133: pp. 505–15, 2010.

[223] Salathe M, Holderby M, Forteza R, Abraham WM, Wanner A, and Conner GE. Isolation and characterization of a peroxidase from the airway. *Am J Respir Cell Mol Biol* 17: pp. 97–105, 1997.

[224] Lieb T, Forteza R, and Salathe M. Hyaluronic acid in cultured ovine tracheal cells and its effect on ciliary beat frequency in vitro. *J Aerosol Med* 13: pp. 231–7, 2000.

[225] Forteza R, Salathe M, Miot F, and Conner GE. Regulated hydrogen peroxide production by Duox in human airway epithelial cells. *Am J Respir Cell Mol Biol* 32: pp. 462–9, 2005.

[226] Lazarowski ER, Sesma JI, Seminario-Vidal L, and Kreda SM. Molecular mechanisms of purine and pyrimidine nucleotide release. *Adv Pharmacol* 61: pp. 221–61, 2011.

[227] Pilette C, Ouadrhiri Y, Godding V, Vaerman JP, and Sibille Y. Lung mucosal immunity: immunoglobulin-A revisited. *Eur Respir J* 18: pp. 571–88, 2001.

[228] Lee CW, Kim TH, Lee HM, Lee SH, Yoo JH, and Kim YS. Upregulation of elafin and cystatin C in the ethmoid sinus mucosa of patients with chronic sinusitis. *Arch Otolaryngol Head Neck Surg* 135: pp. 771–5, 2009.

[229] Hsu AC, Parsons K, Barr I, Lowther S, Middleton D, Hansbro PM, and Wark PA. Critical role of constitutive type I interferon response in bronchial epithelial cell to influenza infection. *PLoS One* 7: p. e32947, 2012.

[230]   Bove PF, and van der Vliet A. Nitric oxide and reactive nitrogen species in airway epithelial signaling and inflammation. *Free Radic Biol Med* 41: pp. 515–27, 2006.

[231]   Hoffmann W. TFF (trefoil factor family) peptides and their potential roles for differentiation processes during airway remodeling. *Curr Med Chem* 14: pp. 2716–9, 2007.

[232]   Kim JK, Kim SS, Rha KW, Kim CH, Cho JH, Lee CH, Lee JG, and Yoon JH. Expression and localization of surfactant proteins in human nasal epithelium. *Am J Physiol* 292: pp. L879–84, 2007.

[233]   Nimishakavi S, Besprozvannaya M, Raymond WW, Craik CS, Gruenert DC, and Caughey GH. Activity and inhibition of prostasin and matriptase on apical and basolateral surfaces of human airway epithelial cells. *Am J Physiol* 303: pp. L97–106, 2012.

[234]   Myerburg MM, McKenna EE, Luke CJ, Frizzell RA, Kleyman TR, and Pilewski JM. Prostasin expression is regulated by airway surface liquid volume and is increased in cystic fibrosis. *Am J Physiol* 294: pp. L932–41, 2008.

[235]   Singh PK, Tack BF, McCray PB, Jr., and Welsh MJ. Synergistic and additive killing by antimicrobial factors found in human airway surface liquid. *Am J Physiol* 279: pp. L799–805, 2000.

[236]   Travis SM, Singh PK, and Welsh MJ. Antimicrobial peptides and proteins in the innate defense of the airway surface. *Curr Opin Immunol* 13: pp. 89–95, 2001.

[237]   Ganz T. Antimicrobial polypeptides in host defense of the respiratory tract. *J Clin Invest* 109: pp. 693–7, 2002.

[238]   Tomasinsig L, and Zanetti M. The cathelicidins—structure, function and evolution. *Curr Protein Pept Sci* 6: pp. 23–34, 2005.

[239]   Cole AM, Ganz T, Liese AM, Burdick MD, Liu L, and Strieter RM. Cutting edge: IFN-inducible ELR- CXC chemokines display defensin-like antimicrobial activity. *J Immunol* 167: pp. 623–7, 2001.

[240]   Yang D, Chertov O, Bykovskaia SN, Chen Q, Buffo MJ, Shogan J, Anderson M, Schroder JM, Wang JM, Howard OM, and Oppenheim JJ. Beta-defensins: linking innate and adaptive immunity through dendritic and T cell CCR6. *Science* 286: pp. 525–8, 1999.

[241]   Dieu MC, Vanbervliet B, Vicari A, Bridon JM, Oldham E, Ait-Yahia S, Briere F, Zlotnik A, Lebecque S, and Caux C. Selective recruitment of immature and mature dendritic cells by distinct chemokines expressed in different anatomic sites. *J Exp Med* 188: pp. 373–86, 1998.

[242]   Campbell JJ, Hedrick J, Zlotnik A, Siani MA, Thompson DA, and Butcher EC. Chemokines and the arrest of lymphocytes rolling under flow conditions. *Science* 279: pp. 381–4, 1998.

[243]   Golec M. Cathelicidin LL-37: LPS-neutralizing, pleiotropic peptide. *Ann Agric Environ Med* 14: pp. 1–4, 2007.

[244]   Barlow PG, Beaumont PE, Cosseau C, Mackellar A, Wilkinson TS, Hancock RE, Has-
lett C, Govan JR, Simpson AJ, and Davidson DJ. The human cathelicidin LL-37 preferentially promotes apoptosis of infected airway epithelium. *Am J Respir Cell Mol Biol* 43:
pp. 692–702, 2010.

[245]   Scott A, Weldon S, and Taggart CC. SLPI and elafin: multifunctional antiproteases of the
WFDC family. *Biochem Soc Trans* 39: pp. 1437–40, 2011.

[246]   Johnson EE, and Wessling-Resnick M. Iron metabolism and the innate immune response
to infection. *Microbes Infect* 14: pp. 207–16, 2012.

[247]   Chan YR, Liu JS, Pociask DA, Zheng M, Mietzner TA, Berger T, Mak TW, Clifton MC,
Strong RK, Ray P, and Kolls JK. Lipocalin 2 is required for pulmonary host defense against
Klebsiella infection. *J Immunol* 182: pp. 4947–56, 2009.

[248]   Fischer H. Mechanisms and function of DUOX in epithelia of the lung. *Antioxid Redox
Signal* 11: pp. 2453–65, 2009.

[249]   Thomas EL, and Aune TM. Lactoperoxidase, peroxide, thiocyanate antimicrobial system:
correlation of sulfhydryl oxidation with antimicrobial action. *Infect Immun* 20: pp. 456–63,
1978.

[250]   Lauer ME, Erzurum SC, Mukhopadhyay D, Vasanji A, Drazba J, Wang A, Fulop C,
and Hascall VC. Differentiated murine airway epithelial cells synthesize a leukocyte-
adhesive hyaluronan matrix in response to endoplasmic reticulum stress. *J Biol Chem* 283:
pp. 26283–96, 2008.

[251]   Forteza R, Lieb T, Aoki T, Savani RC, Conner GE, and Salathe M. Hyaluronan serves a
novel role in airway mucosal host defense. *FASEB J* 15: pp. 2179–86, 2001.

[252]   Proud D, and Vio CP. Localization of immunoreactive tissue kallikrein in human trachea.
Am J Respir Cell Mol Biol 8: pp. 16–9, 1993.

[253]   Bingle L, and Bingle CD. Distribution of human PLUNC/BPI fold-containing (BPIF)
proteins. *Biochem Soc Trans* 39: pp. 1023–7, 2011.

[254]   Gakhar L, Bartlett JA, Penterman J, Mizrachi D, Singh PK, Mallampalli RK, Ramaswamy
S, and McCray PB, Jr. PLUNC is a novel airway surfactant protein with anti-biofilm activity. *PLoS One* 5: p. e9098, 2010.

[255]   Garcia-Caballero A, Rasmussen JE, Gaillard E, Watson MJ, Olsen JC, Donaldson SH,
Stutts MJ, and Tarran R. SPLUNC1 regulates airway surface liquid volume by protecting
ENaC from proteolytic cleavage. *Proc Natl Acad Sci USA* 106: pp. 11412–7, 2009.

[256]   Lakind JS, Holgate ST, Ownby DR, Mansur AH, Helms PJ, Pyatt D, and Hays SM. A
critical review of the use of Clara cell secretory protein (CC16) as a biomarker of acute or
chronic pulmonary effects. *Biomarkers* 12: pp. 445–67, 2007.

[257]   Kasper M, Sims G, Koslowski R, Kuss H, Thuemmler M, Fehrenbach H, and Auten RL.

Increased surfactant protein D in rat airway goblet and Clara cells during ovalbumin-induced allergic airway inflammation. *Clin Exp Allergy* 32: pp. 1251–8, 2002.

[258] Kuroki Y, Takahashi M, and Nishitani C. Pulmonary collectins in innate immunity of the lung. *Cell Microbiol* 9: pp. 1871–9, 2007.

[259] Garcia-Verdugo I, Descamps D, Chignard M, Touqui L, and Sallenave JM. Lung protease/anti-protease network and modulation of mucus production and surfactant activity. *Biochimie* 92: pp. 1608–17, 2010.

[260] Saitoh H, Masuda T, Shimura S, Fushimi T, and Shirato K. Secretion and gene expression of secretory leukocyte protease inhibitor by human airway submucosal glands. *Am J Physiol* 280: pp. L79–87, 2001.

[261] Thim L, Madsen F, and Poulsen SS. Effect of trefoil factors on the viscoelastic properties of mucus gels. *Eur J Clin Invest* 32: pp. 519–27, 2002.

[262] Kaetzel CS. The polymeric immunoglobulin receptor: bridging innate and adaptive immune responses at mucosal surfaces. *Immunol Rev* 206: pp. 83–99, 2005.

[263] Goodman MR, Link DW, Brown WR, and Nakane PK. Ultrastructural evidence of trasport of secretory IgA across bronchial epithelium. *Am Rev Respir Dis* 123: pp. 115–9, 1981.

[264] Polosukhin VV, Cates JM, Lawson WE, Zaynagetdinov R, Milstone AP, Massion PP, Ocak S, Ware LB, Lee JW, Bowler RP, Kononov AV, Randell SH, and Blackwell TS. Bronchial secretory immunoglobulin a deficiency correlates with airway inflammation and progression of chronic obstructive pulmonary disease. *Am J Respir Crit Care Med* 184: pp. 317–27, 2011.

[265] Davis CW, and Lazarowski E. Coupling of airway ciliary activity and mucin secretion to mechanical stresses by purinergic signaling. *Respir Physiol Neurobiol* 163: pp. 208–13, 2008.

[266] Huang P, Gilmore E, Kultgen P, Barnes P, Milgram S, and Stutts MJ. Local regulation of cystic fibrosis transmembrane regulator and epithelial sodium channel in airway epithelium. *Proc Am Thorac Soc* 1: pp. 33–7, 2004.

[267] Button B, Picher M, and Boucher RC. Differential effects of cyclic and constant stress on ATP release and mucociliary transport by human airway epithelia. *J Physiol* 580: pp. 577–92, 2007.

[268] Okada SF, Zhang L, Kreda SM, Abdullah LH, Davis CW, Pickles RJ, Lazarowski ER, and Boucher RC. Coupled nucleotide and mucin hypersecretion from goblet-cell metaplastic human airway epithelium. *Am J Respir Cell Mol Biol* 45: pp. 253–60, 2011.

[269] Proud D, and Leigh R. Epithelial cells and airway diseases. *Immunol Rev* 242: pp. 186–204, 2011.

[270] Holtzman MJ. Arachidonic acid metabolism in airway epithelial cells. *Ann Rev Physiol* 54: pp. 303–29, 1992.

[271] Al-Bazzaz FJ, Yadava VP, and Westenfelder C. Modification of Na and Cl⁻ transport in canine tracheal mucosa by prostaglandins. *Am J Physiol* 240: pp. F101–5, 1981.

[272] Leikauf GD, Ueki IF, Widdicombe JH, and Nadel JA. Alteration of chloride secretion across canine tracheal epithelium by lipoxygenase products of arachidonic acid. *Am J Physiol* 250: pp. F47–53, 1986.

[273] Goldman DW, Gifford LA, Marotti T, Koo CH, and Goetzl EJ. Molecular and cellular properties of human polymorphonuclear leukocyte receptors for leukotriene B4. *Fed Proc* 46: pp. 200–3, 1987.

[274] Back M. Leukotriene receptors: crucial components in vascular inflammation. *Scientific World J* 7: pp. 1422–39, 2007.

[275] Jacobs ER, and Zeldin DC. The lung HETEs (and EETs) up. *Am J Physiol* 280: pp. H1–10, 2001.

[276] Folkerts G, and Nijkamp FP. Airway epithelium: more than just a barrier! *Trends Pharmacol* 19: 3 pp. 34–41, 1998.

[277] Hay DW, Van Scott MR, and Muccitelli RM. Characterization of endothelin release from guinea-pig tracheal epithelium: influence of proinflammatory mediators including major basic protein. *Pulm Pharmacol Ther* 10: pp. 189–98, 1997.

[278] Linsdell P, and Hanrahan JW. Glutathione permeability of CFTR. *Am J Physiol* 275: pp. C323–6, 1998.

[279] Proskocil BJ, Sekhon HS, Jia Y, Savchenko V, Blakely RD, Lindstrom J, and Spindel ER. Acetylcholine is an autocrine or paracrine hormone synthesized and secreted by airway bronchial epithelial cells. *Endocrinology* 145: pp. 2498–506, 2004.

[280] Webber SE, and Widdicombe JG. The transport of albumin across the ferret *in vitro* whole trachea. *J Physiol* 408: pp. 457–72, 1989.

[281] Johnson LG, Cheng PW, and Boucher RC. Albumin absorption by canine bronchial epithelium. *J Appl Physiol* 66: pp. 2772–7, 1989.

[282] Sekizawa K, Tamaoki J, Graf PD, Basbaum CB, Borson DB, and Nadel JA. Enkephalinase inhibitor potentiates mammalian tachykinin-induced contraction in ferret trachea. *J Pharmacol Exp Ther* 243: pp. 1211–7, 1987.

[283] Ohrui T, Yamauchi K, Sekizawa K, Ohkawara T, Maeyama K, Sasaki M, Takemura M, Wada H, Watanabe T, Sasaki H, and Takishima T. Histamine N-methyltransferase controls the contractile response of guinea pig trachea to histamine. *J Pharm Exp Ther* 261: pp. 1268–72, 1992.

[284] Fischer H. Function of proton channels in lung epithelia. *WIREs Membr Transp Signal* doi: 10.1002/wmts.17, 2011.

[285] Fischer H, and Widdicombe JH. Mechanisms of acid and base secretion by the airway epithelium. *J Membr Biol* 211: pp. 139–50, 2006.

[286] Pezzulo AA, Tang XX, Hoegger MJ, Alaiwa MH, Ramachandran S, Moninger TO, Karp PH, Wohlford-Lenane CL, Haagsman HP, van Eijk M, Banfi B, Horswill AR, Stoltz DA, McCray PB, Jr., Welsh MJ, and Zabner J. Reduced airway surface pH impairs bacterial killing in the porcine cystic fibrosis lung. *Nature* 487: pp. 109–13, 2012.

[287] Jayaraman S, Song Y, and Verkman AS. Airway surface liquid pH in well-differentiated airway epithelial cell cultures and mouse trachea. *Am J Physiol* 281: pp. C1504–11, 2001.

[288] Song Y, Salinas D, Nielson DW, and Verkman AS. Hyperacidity of secreted fluid from submucosal glands in early cystic fibrosis. *Am J Physiol* 290: pp. C741–9, 2006.

[289] Coakley RD, Grubb BR, Paradiso AM, Gatzy JT, Johnson LG, Kreda SM, O'Neal WK, and Boucher RC. Abnormal surface liquid pH regulation by cultured cystic fibrosis bronchial epithelium. *Proc Natl Acad Sci USA* 100: pp. 16083–8, 2003.

[290] Devor DC, Singh AK, Lambert LC, DeLuca A, Frizzell RA, and Bridges RJ. Bicarbonate and chloride secretion in Calu-3 human airway epithelial cells. *J Gen Physiol* 113: pp. 743–60, 1999.

[291] Ballard ST, Trout L, Garrison J, and Inglis SK. Ionic mechanism of forskolin-induced liquid secretion by porcine bronchi. *Am J Physiol* 290: pp. L97–104, 2006.

[292] Welsh MJ, Smith PL, and Frizzell RA. Chloride secretion by canine tracheal epithelium II. The cellular electrical potential profile. *J Membr Biol* 70: pp. 227–38, 1982.

[293] Welsh MJ. Intracellular chloride activities in canine tracheal epithelium. Direct evidence for sodium-coupled chloride accumulation in chloride-secreting epithelium. *J Clin Invest* 71: pp. 1392–401, 1983.

[294] Paradiso AM, Coakley RD, and Boucher RC. Polarized distribution of HCO_3^- transport in human normal and cystic fibrosis nasal epithelia. *J Physiol* 548: pp. 203–18, 2003.

[295] Illek B, Tam AW, Fischer H, and Machen TE. Anion selectivity of apical membrane conductance of Calu 3 human airway epithelium. *Pflugers Archiv* 437: pp. 812–22, 1999.

[296] Rajagopal M, Fischer H, and Widdicombe JH. Hormonal and purinergic stimulation of bicarbonate secretion in oviducts of rhesus monkey. *Am J Physiol* 295: pp. E55–62, 2008.

[297] Chang MH, Plata C, Zandi-Nejad K, Sindic A, Sussman CR, Mercado A, Broumand V, Raghuram V, Mount DB, and Romero MF. Slc26a9—anion exchanger, channel and Na^+ transporter. *J Memb Biol* 228: pp. 125–40, 2009.

[298] Inglis SK, Wilson SM, and Olver RE. Secretion of acid and base equivalents by intact distal airways. *Am J Physiol* 284: pp. L855–62, 2003.

[299] Fischer H, Widdicombe JH, and Illek B. Acid secretion and proton conductance in human airway epithelium. *Am J Physiol* 282: pp. C736–43, 2002.

[300] Iovannisci D, Illek B, and Fischer H. Function of the HVCN1 proton channel in airway epithelia and a naturally occurring mutation, M91T. *J Gen Physiol* 136: pp. 35–46, 2010.

[301] Decoursey TE. Voltage-gated proton channels and other proton transfer pathways. *Physiol Rev* 83: pp. 475–579, 2003.

[302] Paradiso AM. Identification of Na^+-H^+ exchange in human normal and cystic fibrotic ciliated airway epithelium. *Am J Physiol* 262: pp. L757–64, 1992.

[303] Knowles MR, Buntin WH, Bromberg PA, Gatzy JT, and Boucher RC. Measurements of transepithelial electric potential difference in the trachea and bronchi of human subjects in vivo. *Am Rev Resp Dis* 126: pp. 108–12, 1982.

[304] Knowles MR, Gatzy JT, and Boucher RC. Increased bioelectric potential differences across respiratory epithelia in cystic fibrosis. *N Engl J Med* 305: pp. 1489–95, 1981.

[305] Boucher RC, Bromberg PA, and Gatzy JT. Airway transepithelial electric potential in vivo: species and regional differences. *J Appl Physiol* 48: pp. 169–76, 1980.

[306] Yamaya M, Finkbeiner WE, Chun SY, and Widdicombe JH. Differentiated structure and function of cultures from human tracheal epithelium. *Am J Physiol* 262: pp. L713–24, 1992.

[307] Kondo M, Finkbeiner WE, and Widdicombe JH. Cultures of bovine tracheal epithelium with differentiated ultrastructure and ion transport. *In Vitro* 29A: pp. 19–24, 1993.

[308] Takahashi M, Freed AN, and Croxton TL. Scaling of transepithelial potential difference in the mammalian trachea. *Respir Physiol* 99: pp. 19–27, 1995.

[309] Melon J. Activite secretoire de la muquese nasale. *Acta Otorhinolaryngol Belg* 22: 11–244, 1968.

[310] Ussing HH, and Zerahn K. Active transport of sodium as the source of electric current in short-circuited isolated frog skin. *Acta Physiol Scand* 23: pp. 110–27, 1951.

[311] Moessinger AC, Harding R, Adamson TM, Singh M, and Kiu GT. Role of lung fluid volume in growth and maturation of the fetal sheep lung. *J Clin Invest* 86: pp. 1270–7, 1990.

[312] Widdicombe JH. Development of fluid transport across pulmonary epithelia. In: *The Lung: Development, Aging and the Environment*, edited by Harding R, Pinkerton KE and Plopper CG. Amsterdam: Elsevier, 2004, pp. 119–29.

[313] Langridge-Smith JE, Rao MC, and Field M. Chloride and sodium transport across bovine tracheal epithelium: effects of secretagogues and indomethacin. *Pfluegers Arch* 402: pp. 42–7, 1984.

[314] Boucher RC, Stutts MJ, Knowles MR, Cantley L, and Gatzy JT. Na^+ transport in cystic fibrosis respiratory epithelia. Abnormal basal rate and response to adenylate cyclase activation. *J Clin Invest* 78: pp. 1245–52, 1986.

[315] Cotton CU, Lawson EE, Boucher RC, and Gatzy JT. Bioelectric properties and ion transport of airways excised from adult and fetal sheep. *J Appl Physiol* 55: pp. 1542–9, 1983.

[316] Gatzy JT, Cotton CU, Boucher RC, Knowles MR, and Gowen CW. Development of epithelial ion transport in fetal and neonatal airways. In: *Physiology of the Fetal and Neonatal Lung*, edited by Walters D, Strang L and Geubelle F. Boston: MTP Press Ltd., 1987, pp. 77–89.

[317] Boucher RC, Stutts MF, and Gatzy JT. Regional differences in bioelectric properties and ion flow in excised canine airways. *J Appl Physiol* 51: pp. 706–14, 1981.

[318] Boucher RC, Narvarte J, Cotton C, Stutts MJ, Knowles MR, Finn AL, and Gatzy JT. Sodium absorption in mammalian airways. In: *Fluid and Electrolyte Abnormalities in Exocrine Glands in Cystic Fibrosis*, edited by Quinton PM, Martinez JR and Hopfer U. San Francisco: San Francisco Press, Inc., 1982, pp. 271–87.

[319] Phipps RJ, Denas SM, and Wanner A. Antigen stimulates glycoprotein secretion and alters ion fluxes in sheep trachea. *J Appl Physiol* 55: pp. 1593–602, 1983.

[320] Al-Bazzaz FJ. Regulation of Na^+ and Cl^- transport in sheep distal airways. *Am J Physiol* 267: pp. L193–8, 1994.

[321] Ropke M, Carstens S, Holm M, and Frederiksen O. Ion transport mechanisms in native rabbit nasal airway epithelium. *Am J Physiol* 271: pp. L637–45, 1996.

[322] Jarnigan F, Davis JD, Bromberg PA, Gatzy JT, and Boucher RC. Bioelectric properties and ion transport of excised rabbit trachea. *J Appl Physiol* 55: pp. 1884–92, 1983.

[323] Corrales RJ, Coleman DL, Jacoby DB, Leikauf GD, Hahn HL, Nadel JA, and Widdicombe JH. Ion transport across cat and ferret tracheal epithelia. *J Appl Physiol* 61: pp. 1065–70, 1986.

[324] Olver R, Davis B, Marin M, and Nadel JA. Active transport of Na^+ and Cl^- across the canine tracheal epithelium in vitro. *Am Rev Respir Dis* 112: pp. 811–5, 1975.

[325] Tessier GJ, Traynor TR, Kannan MS, and O'Grady SM. Mechanisms of sodium and chloride transport across equine tracheal epithelium. *Am J Physiol* 259: pp. L459–67, 1990.

[326] Welsh MJ. Electrolyte transport by airway epithelia. *Physiol Rev* 67: pp. 1143–84, 1987.

[327] Shorofsky SR, Field M, and Fozzard HA. Mechanism of Cl^- secretion in canine trachea: Changes in intracellular chloride activity with secretion. *J Memb Biol* 81: pp. 1–8, 1984.

[328] Widdicombe JH, Basbaum CB, and Yee JY. Localization of Na pumps in the tracheal epithelium of the dog. *J Cell Biol* 82: pp. 380–90, 1979.

[329] Welsh MJ. Evidence for a basolateral membrane potassium conductance in canine tracheal epithelium. *Am J Physiol* 244: pp. C377–84, 1983.

[330] Koefoed-Johnsen V, and Ussing HH. The nature of the frog skin potential. *Acta Physiol Scand* 42: pp. 298–308, 1958.

[331] Shorofsky SR, Field M, and Fozzard HA. Changes in intracellular sodium with chloride secretion in dog tracheal epithelium. *Am J Physiol* 250: pp. C646–50, 1986.

[332] Smith PL, and Frizzell RA. Chloride secretion by canine tracheal epithelium: IV. Basolateral membrane K permeability parallels secretion rate. *J Membr Biol* 77: pp. 187–99, 1984.

[333] Willumsen NJ, and Boucher RC. Sodium transport and intracellular sodium activity in cultured human nasal epithelium. *Am J Physiol* 261: pp. C319–31, 1991.

[334] Willumsen NJ, Davis CW, and Boucher RC. Intracellular Cl$^-$ activity and cellular Cl$^-$ pathways in cultured human airway epithelium. *Am J Physiol* 256: pp. C1033–44, 1989.

[335] Welsh MJ, Smith PL, and Frizzell RA. Chloride secretion by canine tracheal epithelium: III. Membrane resistances and electromotive forces. *J Memb Biol* 71: pp. 209–18, 1983.

[336] Willumsen NJ, and Boucher RC. Shunt resistance and ion permeabilities in normal and cystic fibrosis airway epithelia. *Am J Physiol*: pp. C1054–63, 1989.

[337] Shorofsky SR, Field M, and Fozzard H. Electrophysiology of Cl$^-$ secretion in canine trachea. *J Memb Biol* 72: pp. 105–16, 1983.

[338] Boucher RC, and Gatzy JT. Characteristics of sodium transport by excised rabbit trachea. *J Appl Physiol* 55: pp. 1877–83, 1983.

[339] Al-Bazzaz F. Role of cyclic AMP in regulation of chloride secretion by canine tracheal mucosa. *Am Rev Respir Dis* 123: pp. 295–8, 1981.

[340] Uyekubo SN, Fischer H, Maminishkis A, Illek B, Miller SS, and Widdicombe JH. cAMP-dependent absorption of chloride across airway epithelium. *Am J Physiol* 275: pp. L1219–27, 1998.

[341] Jayaraman S, Song Y, Vetrivel L, Shankar L, and Verkman AS. Noninvasive in vivo fluorescence measurement of airway-surface liquid depth, salt concentration, and pH. *J Clin Investig* 107: pp. 317–24, 2001.

[342] Schultz SG. Homocellular regulatory mechanisms in sodium-transporting epithelia: avoidance of extinction by 'flush through'. *Am J Physiol* 241: pp. F579–90, 1981.

[343] Haas M, McBrayer DG, and Yankaskas JR. Dual mechanisms for Na-K-Cl cotransport regulation in airway epithelial cells. *Am J Physiol* 264: pp. C189–200, 1993.

[344] Haas M, McBrayer D, and Lytle C. [Cl$^-$]$_i$-dependent phosphorylation of the Na-K-Cl cotransport protein of dog tracheal epithelial cells. *J Biol Chem* 270: pp. 28955–61, 1995.

[345] Thomas RC. Membrane current and intracellular sodium changes in a snail neurone during extrusion of injected sodium. *J Physiol* 201: pp. 495–514, 1969.

[346] Welsh MJ. Basolateral membrane potassium conductance is independent of sodium pump activity and membrane voltage in canine tracheal epithelium. *J Membr Biol* 84: pp. 25–33, 1985.

[347] Yamaya M, Ohrui T, Finkbeiner WE, and Widdicombe JH. Calcium-dependent chloride secretion across cultures of human tracheal surface epithelium and glands. *Am J Physiol* 265: pp. L170–7, 1993.

[348] Namkung W, Finkbeiner WE, and Verkman AS. CFTR-adenylyl cyclase I association responsible for UTP activation of CFTR in well-differentiated primary human bronchial cell cultures. *Mol Biol Cell* 21: pp. 2639–48, 2010.

[349] Widdicombe JH, Welsh MJ, and Finkbeiner WE. Cystic fibrosis decreases the apical membrane chloride permeability of monolayers cultured from cells of tracheal epithelium. *Proc Natl Acad Sci USA* 82: pp. 6167–71, 1985.

[350] Welsh MJ, and Smith AE. Molecular mechanisms of CFTR chloride channel dysfunction in cystic fibrosis. *Cell* 73: pp. 1251–4, 1993.

[351] Welsh MJ, and McCann JD. Intracellular calcium regulates basolateral potassium channels in a chloride-secreting epithelium. *Proc Natl Acad Sci USA* 82: pp. 8823–6, 1985.

[352] Hartzell C, Putzier I, and Arreola J. Calcium-activated chloride channels. *Ann Rev Physiol* 67: pp. 719–58, 2005.

[353] Widdicombe JH. Cystic fibrosis and β-adrenergic response of airway epithelial cell cultures. *Am J Physiol* 251: pp. R818–22, 1986.

[354] Anderson M, and Welsh M. Calcium and cAMP activate different chloride channels in the apical membrane of normal and cystic fibrosis epithelia. *Proc Natl Acad Sci USA* 88: pp. 6003–7, 1991.

[355] Clarke LL, Paradiso AM, Mason SJ, and Boucher RC. Effects of bradykinin on Na^+ and Cl^- transport in human nasal epithelium. *Am J Physiol* 262: pp. C644–55, 1992.

[356] Yang YD, Cho H, Koo JY, Tak MH, Cho Y, Shim WS, Park SP, Lee J, Lee B, Kim BM, Raouf R, Shin YK, and Oh U. TMEM16A confers receptor-activated calcium-dependent chloride conductance. *Nature* 455: pp. 1210–5, 2008.

[357] Caputo A, Caci E, Ferrera L, Pedemonte N, Barsanti C, Sondo E, Pfeffer U, Ravazzolo R, Zegarra-Moran O, and Galietta LJ. TMEM16A, a membrane protein associated with calcium-dependent chloride channel activity. *Science* 322: pp. 590–4, 2008.

[358] Schroeder BC, Cheng T, Jan YN, and Jan LY. Expression cloning of TMEM16A as a calcium-activated chloride channel subunit. *Cell* 134: pp. 1019–29, 2008.

[359] Ousingsawat J, Martins JR, Schreiber R, Rock JR, Harfe BD, and Kunzelmann K. Loss of TMEM16A causes a defect in epithelial Ca^{2+}-dependent chloride transport. *J Biol Chem* 284: pp. 28698–703, 2009.

[360] Rock JR, O'Neal WK, Gabriel SE, Randell SH, Harfe BD, Boucher RC, and Grubb BR. Transmembrane protein 16A (TMEM16A) is a Ca^{2+}-regulated Cl^- secretory channel in mouse airways. *J Biol Chem* 284: pp. 14875–80, 2009.

[361] Namkung W, Phuan PW, and Verkman AS. TMEM16A inhibitors reveal TMEM16A as a minor component of calcium-activated chloride channel conductance in airway and intestinal epithelial cells. *J Biol Chem* 286: pp. 2365–74, 2011.

[362] Dorwart MR, Shcheynikov N, Yang D, and Muallem S. The solute carrier 26 family of proteins in epithelial ion transport. *Physiology (Bethesda)* 23: pp. 104–14, 2008.

[363] Dorwart MR, Shcheynikov N, Wang Y, Stippec S, and Muallem S. SLC26A9 is a Cl^- channel regulated by the WNK kinases. *J Physiol* 584: pp. 333–45, 2007.

[364]   Lohi H, Kujala M, Makela S, Lehtonen E, Kestila M, Saarialho-Kere U, Markovich D, and Kere J. Functional characterization of three novel tissue-specific anion exchangers SLC26A7, -A8, and -A9. *J Biol Chem* 277: pp. 14246–54, 2002.

[365]   Bertrand CA, Zhang R, Pilewski JM, and Frizzell RA. SLC26A9 is a constitutively active, CFTR-regulated anion conductance in human bronchial epithelia. *J Gen Physiol* 133: pp. 421–38, 2009.

[366]   Benos DJ. Amiloride: a molecular probe of sodium transport in tissues and cells. *Am J Physiol* 242: pp. C131–45, 1982.

[367]   Canessa CM, Schild L, Buell G, Thorens B, Gautschi I, Horisberger JD, and Rossier BC. Amiloride-sensitive epithelial Na$^+$ channel is made of three homologous subunits. *Nature* 367: pp. 463–67, 1994.

[368]   Mueller GM, Kashlan OB, Bruns JB, Maarouf AB, Aridor M, Kleyman TR, and Hughey RP. Epithelial sodium channel exit from the endoplasmic reticulum is regulated by a signal within the carboxyl cytoplasmic domain of the alpha subunit. *J Biol Chem* 282: pp. 33475–83, 2007.

[369]   Helms MN, Self J, Bao HF, Job LC, Jain L, and Eaton DC. Dopamine activates amiloride-sensitive sodium channels in alveolar type I cells in lung slice preparations. *Am J Physiol* 291: pp. L610–8, 2006.

[370]   Burch LH, Talbot CR, Knowles MR, Canessa CM, Rossier BC, and Boucher RC. Relative expression of the human epithelial Na$^+$ channel subunits in normal and cystic fibrosis airways. *Am J Physiol* 269: pp. C511–8, 1995.

[371]   Farman N, Talbot CR, Boucher R, Fay M, Canessa C, Rossier B, and Bonvalet JP. Non-coordinated expression of alpha-, beta-, and gamma-subunit mRNAs of epithelial Na$^+$ channel along rat respiratory tract. *Am J Physiol* 272: pp. C131–41, 1997.

[372]   Matsushita K, McCray PB, Jr., Sigmund RD, Welsh MJ, and Stokes JB. Localization of epithelial sodium channel subunit mRNAs in adult rat lung by in situ hybridization. *Am J Physiol* 271: pp. L332–9, 1996.

[373]   Zhao RZ, Nie HG, Su XF, Han DY, Lee A, Huang Y, Chang Y, Matalon S, and Ji HL. Characterization of a novel splice variant of delta ENaC subunit in human lungs. *Am J Physiol*, 2012.

[374]   Bangel-Ruland N, Sobczak K, Christmann T, Kentrup D, Langhorst H, Kusche-Vihrog K, and Weber WM. Characterization of the epithelial sodium channel delta-subunit in human nasal epithelium. *Am J Respir Cell Mol Biol* 42: pp. 498–505, 2010.

[375]   Gaillard EA, Kota P, Gentzsch M, Dokholyan NV, Stutts MJ, and Tarran R. Regulation of the epithelial Na$^+$ channel and airway surface liquid volume by serine proteases. *Pflugers Arch* 460: pp. 1–17, 2010.

[376]   Myerburg MM, Butterworth MB, McKenna EE, Peters KW, Frizzell RA, Kleyman TR,

and Pilewski JM. Airway surface liquid volume regulates ENaC by altering the serine protease-protease inhibitor balance: a mechanism for sodium hyperabsorption in cystic fibrosis. *J Biol Chem* 281: pp. 27942–9, 2006.

[377] Stokes JB, and Sigmund RD. Regulation of rENaC mRNA by dietary NaCl and steroids: organ, tissue, and steroid heterogeneity. *Am J Physiol* 274: pp. C1699–707, 1998.

[378] Bardou O, Trinh NT, and Brochiero E. Molecular diversity and function of K$^+$ channels in airway and alveolar epithelial cells. *Am J Physiol* 296: pp. L145–55, 2009.

[379] Mall M, Wissner A, Schreiber R, Kuehr J, Seydewitz HH, Brandis M, Greger R, and Kunzelmann K. Role of K(V)LQT1 in cyclic adenosine monophosphate-mediated Cl$^-$ secretion in human airway epithelia. *Am J Respir Cell Mol Biol* 23: pp. 283–9, 2000.

[380] Grahammer F, Warth R, Barhanin J, Bleich M, and Hug MJ. The small conductance K$^+$ channel, KCNQ1: expression, function, and subunit composition in murine trachea. *J Biol Chem* 276: pp. 42268–75, 2001.

[381] Namkung W, Song Y, Mills AD, Padmawar P, Finkbeiner WE, and Verkman AS. In situ measurement of airway surface liquid K$^+$ using a ratioable K$^+$-sensitive fluorescent dye. *J Biol Chem* 284: pp. 15916–26, 2009.

[382] Mall M, Gonska T, Thomas J, Schreiber R, Seydewitz HH, Kuehr J, Brandis M, and Kunzelmann K. Modulation of Ca^{2+}-activated Cl$^-$ secretion by basolateral K$^+$ channels in human normal and cystic fibrosis airway epithelia. *Pediatr Res* 53: pp. 608–18, 2003.

[383] Kunzelmann K, Pavenstadt H, Beck C, Unal O, Emmrich P, Arndt HJ, and Greger R. Characterization of potassium channels in respiratory cells. I. General properties. *Pflugers Arch* 414: pp. 291–6, 1989.

[384] Manzanares D, Gonzalez C, Ivonnet P, Chen RS, Valencia-Gattas M, Conner GE, Larsson HP, and Salathe M. Functional apical large conductance, Ca^{2+}-activated, and voltage-dependent K$^+$ channels are required for maintenance of airway surface liquid volume. *J Biol Chem* 286: pp. 19830–9, 2011.

[385] Welsh MJ. Energetics of chloride secretion in canine tracheal epithelium: comparison of the metabolic cost of chloride transport with the metabolic cost of sodium transport. *J Clin Invest* 74: pp. 262–8, 1984.

[386] Fong P, Chao AC, and Widdicombe JH. Potassium dependence of Na-Cl cotransport in dog tracheal epithelium. *Am J Physiol* 261: pp. L290–5, 1991.

[387] Haas M, Johnson LG, and Boucher RC. Regulation of Na-K-Cl cotransport in cultured canine airway epithelia: a [^{3}H]bumetanide binding study. *Am J Physiol* 259: pp. C557–69, 1990.

[388] Haas M, and McBrayer DG. Na-K-Cl cotransport in nystatin-treated tracheal cells: regulation by isoproterenol, apical UTP, and [Cl$^-$]$_i$. *Am J Physiol* 266: pp. C1440–52, 1994.

[389] Treharne KJ, Marshall LJ, and Mehta A. A novel chloride-dependent GTP-utilizing

protein kinase in plasma membranes from human respiratory epithelium. *Am J Physiol* 267: pp. L592–601, 1994.

[390] Russell JM. Sodium-potassium-chloride cotransport. *Physiol Rev* 80: pp. 211–76, 2000.

[391] Liedtke CM. Calcium and α-adrenergic regulation of Na-Cl(K) contransport in rabbit tracheal epithelial cells. *Am J Physiol* 259: pp. L66–72, 1990.

[392] Liedtke CM. Bumetanide-sensitive NaCl uptake in rabbit tracheal epithelial cells is stimulated by neurohormones and hypertonicity. *Am J Physiol* 262: pp. L621–7, 1992.

[393] Liedtke CM, and Cole TS. Antisense oligonucleotide to PKC-epsilon alters cAMP-dependent stimulation of CFTR in Calu-3 cells. *Am J Physiol* 275: pp. C1357–64, 1998.

[394] Smith L, Smallwood N, Altman A, and Liedtke CM. PKCdelta acts upstream of SPAK in the activation of NKCC1 by hyperosmotic stress in human airway epithelial cells. *J Biol Chem* 283: pp. 22147–56, 2008.

[395] Widdicombe JH, Basbaum CB, and Highland E. Sodium-pump density of cells from dog tracheal mucosa. *Am J Physiol* 248: pp. C389–98, 1985.

[396] Fischer H, Illek B, Finkbeiner WE, and Widdicombe JH. Basolateral Cl⁻ channels in primary airway epithelial cultures. *Am J Physiol* 292: pp. L1432–43, 2007.

[397] Itani OA, Lamb FS, Melvin JE, and Welsh MJ. Basolateral chloride current in human airway epithelia. *Am J Physiol* 293: pp. L991–9, 2007.

[398] Clarke LL, and Boucher RC. Chloride secretory response to extracellular ATP in human normal and cystic fibrosis nasal epithelia. *Am J Physiol* 263: pp. C348–56, 1992.

[399] Widdicombe JH. Ion and fluid transport by airway epithelium. In: *Airway Secretion: Physiological Bases for the Control of Mucus Hypersecretion*, edited by Takishima T and Shimura S. New York: Marcel Dekker, Inc., 1993, pp. 399–431.

[400] Pratt AD, Clancy G, and Welsh MJ. Mucosal adenosine stimulates chloride secretion in canine tracheal epithelium. *Am J Physiol* 251: pp. C167–74, 1986.

[401] Xie W, Fisher JT, Lynch TJ, Luo M, Evans TI, Neff TL, Zhou W, Zhang Y, Ou Y, Bunnett NW, Russo AF, Goodheart MJ, Parekh KR, Liu X, and Engelhardt JF. CGRP induction in cystic fibrosis airways alters the submucosal gland progenitor cell niche in mice. *J Clin Invest* 121: pp. 3144–58, 2011.

[402] Al-Bazzaz FJ, and Cheng E. Effect of catecholamines on ion transport in dog tracheal epithelium. *J Appl Physiol* 47: pp. 397–403, 1979.

[403] Nathanson I, Widdicombe JH, and Barnes PJ. Effect of vasoactive intestinal peptide on ion transport across dog tracheal epithelium. *J Appl Physiol* 55: pp. 1844–8, 1983.

[404] Smith PL, Welsh MJ, Stoff JS, and Frizzell RA. Chloride secretion by canine tracheal epithelium: I. Role of intracellular cAMP levels. *J Membr Biol* 70: pp. 215–26, 1982.

[405] Mason SJ, Paradiso AM, and Boucher RC. Regulation of transepithelial ion transport and

intracellular calcium by extracellular ATP in human normal and cystic fibrosis airway epithelium. *Br J Pharmacol* 103: pp. 1649–56, 1991.

[406]   Clarke LL, Paradiso AM, and Boucher RC. Histamine-induced Cl⁻ secretion in human nasal epithelium: responses of apical and basolateral membranes. *Am J Physiol* 263: pp. C1190–9, 1992.

[407]   Tessier GJ, Traynor TR, Kannan MS, and O'Grady SM. Mucosal histamine inhibits Na absorption and stimulates Cl⁻ secretion across equine tracheal epithelium. *Am J Physiol* 261: pp. L456–61, 1991.

[408]   Vulliemin P, Durand-Arczynska W, and Durand J. Electrical properties and electrolyte transport in bovine tracheal epithelium: effects of ion substitutions, transport inhibitors and histamine. *Pfluegers Arch* 396: pp. 54–9, 1983.

[409]   Durand J, Durand-Arczynskam W, and Haab P. Volume flow, hydraulic conductivity and electrical properties across bovine tracheal epithlium in vitro: effect of histamine. *Pfluegers Arch* 392: pp. 40–5, 1981.

[410]   Leikauf G, Ueki IF, Nadel JA, and Widdicombe JH. Bradykinin stimulates chloride secretion and prostaglandin E₂ release by canine tracheal epithelium. *Am J Physiol* 248: pp. F48–55, 1985.

[411]   Tamaoki J, Ueki IF, Widdicombe JH, and Nadel JA. Stimulation of Cl⁻ secretion by neurokinin A and neurokinin B in canine tracheal epithelium. *Am Rev Respir Dis* 137: pp. 899–902, 1988.

[412]   Al-Bazzaz FJ, Kelsey J, and Kaage W. Substance P stimulation of chloride secretion by canine tracheal mucosa. *Am Rev Respir Dis* 131: pp. 86–9, 1985.

[413]   Marin MG, Davis B, and Nadel JA. Effect of acetylcholine on Cl⁻ and Na⁺ fluxes across dog tracheal epithelium in vitro. *Am J Physiol* 231: pp. 1546–9, 1976.

[414]   Acevedo M. Effect of acetylcholine on ion transport in sheep tracheal epithelium. *Pflugers Arch* 427: pp. 543–6, 1994.

[415]   Chiyotani A, Tamaoki J, Takeuchi S, Kondo M, Isono K, and Konno K. Stimulation by menthol of Cl⁻ secretion via a Ca²⁺-dependent mechanism in canine airway epithelium. *Br J Pharmacol* 112: pp. 571–5, 1994.

[416]   Clancy JP, McCann JD, and Welsh MJ. Evidence that calcium-dependent activation of airway epithelial chloride channels is not dependent on phosphorylation. *Am J Physiol* 259: pp. L410–4, 1990.

[417]   Cullen JJ, and Welsh MJ. Regulation of sodium absorption by canine tracheal epithelium. *J Clin Invest* 79: pp. 73–9, 1987.

[418]   Devor DC, and Pilewski JM. UTP inhibits Na⁺ absorption in wild-type and DeltaF508 CFTR-expressing human bronchial epithelia. *Am J Physiol* 276: pp. C827–37, 1999.

[419] Inglis SK, Olver RE, and Wilson SM. Differential effects of UTP and ATP on ion transport in porcine tracheal epithelium. *Br J Pharmacol* 130: pp. 367–74, 2000.

[420] Carstairs JR, and Barnes PJ. Visualization of vasoactive intestinal peptide receptors in human and guinea pig lung. *J Pharmacol Exp Ther* 239: pp. 249–55, 1986.

[421] Carstairs R, Nimmo A, and Barnes P. Autoradiographic visualization of β-adrenoceptor subtypes in human lung. *Am Rev Repir Dis* 132: pp. 5541–57, 1985.

[422] Barnes AP, Livera G, Huang P, Sun C, O'Neal WK, Conti M, Stutts MJ, and Milgram SL. Phosphodiesterase 4D forms a cAMP diffusion barrier at the apical membrane of the airway epithelium. *J Biol Chem* 280: pp. 7997–8003, 2005.

[423] Barthelson RA, Jacoby DB, and Widdicombe JH. Regulation of chloride secretion in dog tracheal epithelium by protein kinase C. *Am J Physiol* 253: pp. C802–8, 1987.

[424] Paradiso AM, Ribeiro CM, and Boucher RC. Polarized signaling via purinoceptors in normal and cystic fibrosis airway epithelia. *J Gen Physiol* 117: pp. 53–67, 2001.

[425] Paradiso AM, Mason SJ, Lazarowski ER, and Boucher RC. Membrane-restricted regulation of Ca^{2+} release and influx in polarized epithelia. *Nature* 377: pp. 643–6, 1995.

[426] Ribeiro CM, Paradiso AM, Livraghi A, and Boucher RC. The mitochondrial barriers segregate agonist-induced calcium-dependent functions in human airway epithelia. *J Gen Physiol* 122: pp. 377–87, 2003.

[427] Joris L, and Quinton PM. Filter paper equilibration as a novel technique for in vitro studies of the composition of airway surface fluid. *Am J Physiol* 263: pp. L243–8, 1992.

[428] Clarke LL, Chinet T, and Boucher RC. Extracellular ATP stimulates K^+ secretion across cultured human airway epithelium. *Am J Physiol* 272: pp. L1084–91, 1997.

[429] Fragoso MA, Fernandez V, Forteza R, Randell SH, Salathe M, and Conner GE. Transcellular thiocyanate transport by human airway epithelia. *J Physiol* 561: pp. 183–94, 2004.

[430] Pedemonte N, Caci E, Sondo E, Caputo A, Rhoden K, Pfeffer U, Di Candia M, Bandettini R, Ravazzolo R, Zegarra-Moran O, and Galietta LJ. Thiocyanate transport in resting and IL-4-stimulated human bronchial epithelial cells: role of pendrin and anion channels. *J Immunol* 178: pp. 5144–53, 2007.

[431] Wijkstrom-Frei C, El-Chemaly S, Ali-Rachedi R, Gerson C, Cobas MA, Forteza R, Salathe M, and Conner GE. Lactoperoxidase and human airway host defense. *Am J Respir Cell Mol Biol* 29: pp. 206–12, 2003.

[432] Ashby MT, Carlson AC, and Scott MJ. Redox buffering of hypochlorous acid by thiocyanate in physiologic fluids. *J Am Chem Soc* 126: pp. 15976–7, 2004.

[433] Fischer AJ, Lennemann NJ, Krishnamurthy S, Pocza P, Durairaj L, Launspach JL, Rhein BA, Wohlford-Lenane C, Lorentzen D, Banfi B, and McCray PB, Jr. Enhancement of respiratory mucosal antiviral defenses by the oxidation of iodide. *Am J Respir Cell Mol Biol* 45: pp. 874–81, 2011.

[434]   Al-Bazzaz FJ, and Jayaram T. Calcium secretion in canine tracheal mucosa. *J Appl Physiol* 59: pp. 1191–5, 1985.

[435]   Joris L, and Quinton PM. Evidence for electrogenic Na-glucose cotransport in tracheal epithelium. *Plugers Arch* 65: pp. 118–20, 1989.

[436]   Pezzulo AA, Gutierrez J, Duschner KS, McConnell KS, Taft PJ, Ernst SE, Yahr TL, Rahmouni K, Klesney-tait J, Stoltz DA, and Zabner J. Glucose depletion in the airway surface liquid is essential for sterility of the airways. *PLoS One* 6(1): e16166, 2011.

[437]   Spring KR. Routes and mechanism of fluid transport by epithelia. *Ann Rev Physiol* 60: 105–19, 1998.

[438]   Verkman AS. Aquaporins at a glance. *J Cell Sci* 124: pp. 2107–12, 2011.

[439]   Kreda SM, Gynn MG, Fenstermacher DA, Boucher RC, and Gabriel SE. Expression and localization of epithelial aquaporins in the adult human lung. *Am J Respir Cell Mol Biol* 24: pp. 224–34, 2001.

[440]   Song Y, Jayaraman S, Yang B, Matthay MA, and Verkman AS. Role of aquaporin water channels in airway fluid transport, humidification, and surface liquid hydration. *J Gen Physiol* 117: pp. 573–82, 2001.

[441]   Wine JJ, and Widdicombe JH. Submucosal glands and airway defense. *Physiol Rev* in preparation.

[442]   Cotton CU, Boucher RC, and Gatzy JT. Bioelectric properties and ion transport across excised canine fetal and neonatal airways. *J Applied Physiol* 65: pp. 2367–75, 1988.

[443]   Grubb BR, Schiretz FR, and Boucher RC. Volume transport across tracheal and bronchial airway epithelia in a tubular culture system. *Am J Physiol* 273: pp. C21–9, 1997.

[444]   Zhang Y, Yankaskas J, Wilson J, and Engelhardt JF. *In vivo* analysis of fluid transport in cystic fibrosis airway epithelia of bronchial xenographs. *Am J Physiol* 270: pp. C1326–35, 1996.

[445]   Martens CJ, and Ballard ST. Effects of secretagogues on net and unidirectional liquid fluxes across porcine bronchial airways. *Am J Physiol* 298: pp. L270–6, 2010.

[446]   Smith J, and Welsh M. Fluid and electrolyte transport by cultured human airway epithelia. *J Clin Invest* 91: pp. 1590–7, 1992.

[447]   Kondo M, Tamaoki J, Sakai A, Kamayama S, Kaanoh S, and Konno D. Increased oxidative metabolism in cow tracheal epithelial cells cultured at air-liquid interface. *Am J Respir Cell Mol Biol* 16: pp. 62–8, 1997.

[448]   Rodnight R. Manometric determination of the solubility of oxygen in liquid paraffin, olive oil and silicone fluids. *Biochem J* 57: pp. 661–3, 1954.

[449]   Crews A, Taylor AE, and Ballard ST. Liquid transport properties of porcine tracheal epithelium. *J Appl Physiol* 91: pp. 797–802, 2001.

[450]   Krochmal EM, Ballard ST, Yankaskas JR, Boucher RC, and Gatzy JT. Volume and ion

transport by fetal rat alveolar and tracheal epithelia in submersion culture. *Am J Physiol* 256: pp. F397–407, 1989.

[451] Wiedner G. Method to detect volume flows in the nanoliter range. *Rev Sci Instrum* 47: pp. 775–6, 1976.

[452] Smith JJ, Karp PH, and Welsh MJ. Defective fluid transport by cystic fibrosis airway epithelia. *J Clin Invest* 93: pp. 1307–11, 1994.

[453] Widdicombe J. Relationships among the composition of mucus, epithelial lining liquid, and adhesion of microorganisms. *Am J Respir Crit Care Med* 151: pp. 2088–92, 1995.

[454] Widdicombe JH. Altered NaCl concentration of airway surface liquid in cystic fibrosis. *News Physiol Sci* 14: pp. 126–7, 1999.

[455] Tarran R, Button B, and Boucher RC. Regulation of normal and cystic fibrosis airway surface liquid volume by phasic shear stress. *Ann Rev Physiol* 68: pp. 543–61, 2006.

[456] Widdicombe JH. CFTR and airway pathophysiology. In: *The Cystic Fibrosis Transmembrane Conductance Regulator*, edited by Kirk KL and Dawson DC. New York: Kluwer Academic / Plenum Publishers, 2003, pp. 137–51.

[457] Erjefalt I, and Persson CGA. On the use of absorbing discs to sample mucosal surface liquids. *Clin Exper Allergy* 20: pp. 193–7, 1990.

[458] Landry JS, Landry C, Cowley EA, Govindaraju K, and Eidelman DH. Harvesting airway surface liquid: a comparison of two techniques. *Pediatr Pulmonol* 37: pp. 149–57, 2004.

[459] Knowles MR, Robinson JM, Wood RE, Pue CA, Mentz WM, Wager GC, Gatzy JT, and Boucher RC. Ion composition of airway surface liquid of patients with cystic fibrosis as compared with normal and disease-control subjects. *J Clin Invest* 100: pp. 2588–95, 1997.

[460] Caldwell RA, Grubb BR, Tarran R, Boucher RC, Knowles MR, and Barker PM. In vivo airway surface liquid Cl⁻ analysis with solid-state electrodes. *J Gen Physiol* 119: pp. 3–14, 2002.

[461] Matsui H, Grubb BR, Tarran R, Randell SH, Gatzy JT, Davis CW, and Boucher RC. Evidence for periciliary liquid layer depletion, not abnormal ion composition, in the pathogenesis of cystic fibrosis airways disease. *Cell* 95: pp. 1005–15, 1998.

[462] Zabner J, Smith JJ, Karp PH, Widdicombe JH, and Welsh MJ. Loss of CFTR chloride channels alters salt absorption by cystic fibrosis airway epithelia in vitro. *Mol Cell* 2: pp. 397–403, 1998.

[463] Song Y, Thiagarajah J, and Verkman AS. Sodium and chloride concentrations, pH, and depth of airway surface liquid in distal airways. *J Gen Physiol* 122: pp. 511–9, 2003.

[464] Jayaraman S, Song Y, and Verkman AS. Airway surface liquid osmolality measured using fluorophore-encapsulated liposomes. *J Gen Physiol* 117: pp. 423–30, 2001.

[465] Tarran R, Trout L, Donaldson SH, and Boucher RC. Soluble mediators, not cilia, determine airway surface liquid volume in normal and cystic fibrosis superficial airway epithelia. *J Gen Physiol* 127: pp. 591–604, 2006.

[466] Tarran R, Button B, Picher M, Paradiso AM, Ribeiro CM, Lazarowski ER, Zhang L, Collins PL, Pickles RJ, Fredberg JJ, and Boucher RC. Normal and cystic fibrosis airway surface liquid homeostasis. The effects of phasic shear stress and viral infections. *J Biol Chem* 280: pp. 35751–9, 2005.

[467] Song Y, Namkung W, Nielson DW, Lee JW, Finkbeiner WE, and Verkman AS. Airway surface liquid depth measured in ex vivo fragments of pig and human trachea: dependence on Na^+ and Cl^- channel function. *Am J Physiol* 297: pp. L1131–40, 2009.

[468] Livraghi A, Mall M, Paradiso AM, Boucher RC, and Ribeiro CM. Modelling dysregulated Na^+ absorption in airway epithelial cells with mucosal nystatin treatment. *Am J Respir Cell Mol Biol* 38: pp. 423–34, 2008.

[469] Derichs N, Jin BJ, Song Y, Finkbeiner WE, and Verkman AS. Hyperviscous airway periciliary and mucous liquid layers in cystic fibrosis measured by confocal fluorescence photobleaching. *FASEB J* 25: pp. 2325–32, 2011.

[470] Chen JH, Stoltz DA, Karp PH, Ernst SE, Pezzulo AA, Moninger TO, Rector MV, Reznikov LR, Launspach JL, Chaloner K, Zabner J, and Welsh MJ. Loss of anion transport without increased sodium absorption characterizes newborn porcine cystic fibrosis airway epithelia. *Cell* 143: pp. 911–23, 2010.

[471] Tarran R, Grubb BR, Parsons D, Picher M, Hirsh AJ, Davis CW, and Boucher RC. The CF salt controversy: in vivo observations and therapeutic approaches. *Mol Cell* 8: pp. 149–58, 2001.

[472] Robinson M, and Bye PTB. Mucociliary clearance in cystic fibrsosis. *Ped Pulmonol* 33: pp. 293–306, 2002.

[473] Lansley AB, Sanderson MJ, and Dirksen ER. Control of the beat cycle of respiratory tract cilia by Ca^{2+} and cAMP. *Am J Physiol* 263: pp. L232–42, 1992.

[474] Sanderson MF, and Dirksen ER. Mechanosensitive and beta-adrenergic control of the ciliary beat frequency of mammalian respiratory tract cells in culture. *Am Rev Respir Dis* 139: pp. 432–40, 1989.

[475] Tamaoki J, Kondo M, and Takizawa T. Adenosine-mediated cyclic AMP-dependent inhibition of ciliary activity in rabbit tracheal epithelium. *Am Rev Respir Dis* 139: pp. 441–5, 1989.

[476] Tamaoki J, Kondo M, and Takizawa T. Effect of cAMP on ciliary function in rabbit tracheal epithelial cells. *J Appl Physiol* 66: pp. 1035–9, 1989.

[477] Sanderson MJ, Charles AC, and Dirksen ER. Mechanical stimulation and intercellular

communication increases intracellular Ca^{2+} in epithelial cells. *Cell Reg* 1: pp. 585–96, 1990.

[478]   Boitano S, Dirksen ER, and Sanderson MJ. Intercellular propagation of calcium waves mediated by inositol trisphosphate. *Science* 258: pp. 292–5, 1992.

[479]   Iravani J. Zum Mechanismus der Ortsabhangigkeit der Flimmeraktivitat in Brochialbaum. *Naunyn Schmieder Arch Exp Path Pharm* 264: pp. 248–59, 1969.

[480]   Iravani J, and Melville GN. Mucociliary function in the respiratory tract as influenced by physicochemical factors. *Pharmac Ther B* 2: pp. 471–92, 1976.

[481]   Iravani J. Flimmerbewegung in den intrapulmonalen luftwegen der ratte. *Pflugers Arch* 297: pp. 221–37, 1967.

[482]   Kilburn KH. A hypothesis for pulmonary clearance and its implications. *Am Rev Respir Dis* 98: pp. 449–63, 1968.

[483]   Puchelle E, Zahm JM, and Quemada D. Rheological properties controlling mucociliary frequency and respiratory mucus transport. *Biorheology* 24: pp. 557–63, 1987.

[484]   King M, and Rubin BK. Rheology of airway mucus: relationship with clearance function. In: *Airway Secretion: Physiological Bases for the Control of Mucous Hypersecretion*, edited by Takishima T and Shimura S. New York: Marcel Dekker, 1994, pp. 283–314.

[485]   King M. Physiology of mucus clearance. *Paediatr Respir Rev* 7 Suppl 1: pp. S212–4, 2006.

[486]   Ballard ST, Trout L, Mehta A, and Inglis SK. Liquid secretion inhibitors reduce mucociliary transport in glandular airways. *Am J Physiol* 283: pp. L329–35, 2002.

[487]   Trout L, Townsley MI, Bowden AL, and Ballard ST. Disruptive effects of anion secretion inhibitors on airway mucus morphology in isolated perfused pig lung. *J Physiol* 549: pp. 845–53, 2003.

[488]   Trout L, King M, Feng W, Inglis SK, and Ballard ST. Inhibition of airway liquid secretion and its effect on the physical properties of airway mucus. *Am J Physiol* 274: pp. L258–63, 1998.

[489]   Van As A, and Webster I. The morphology of mucus in mammalian pulmonary airways. *Env Res* 7: pp. 1–12, 1974.

[490]   Sears PR, Davis CW, Chua M, and Sheehan JK. Mucociliary interactions and mucus dynamics in ciliated bronchial epithelial cultures. *Am J Physiol* 301: pp. L181–6, 2011.

[491]   Widdicombe JH, Shen B-Q, and Finkbeiner WE. Structure and function of human airway mucous glands in health and disease. *Adv Struct Biol* 3: pp. 225–41, 1994.

[492]   Ballard ST, and Inglis SK. Liquid secretion properties of airway submucosal glands. *J Physiol* 556: pp. 1–10, 2004.

[493]   Meyrick B, Sturgess JM, and Reid L. A reconstruction of the duct system and secretory tubules of the human bronchial submucosal gland. *Thorax* 24: pp. 729–36, 1969.

[494]   Inglis SK, Corboz MR, Taylor AE, and Ballard ST. In situ visualization of bronchial sub-

mucosal glands and their secretory response to acetylcholine. *Am J Physiol* 272: pp. L203–10, 1997.

[495] Ballard ST, Schepens SM, Falcone JC, Meininger GA, and Taylor AE. Regional bioelectric properties of porcine airways epithelium. *J Appl Physiol* 73: pp. 2021–7, 1992.

[496] Mariassy AT, and Plopper CG. Tracheobronchial epithelium of the sheep: 1. Quantitative light-microscopic study of epithelial cell abundance, and distribution. *Anat Rec* 205: pp. 263–75, 1983.

[497] Borthwick DW, West JD, Keighren MA, Flockhart JH, Innes BA, and Dorin JR. Murine submucosal glands are clonally derived and show a cystic fibrosis gene-dependent distribution pattern. *Am J Respir Cell Mol Biol* 20: pp. 1181–9, 1999.

[498] Ianowski JP, Choi JY, Wine JJ, and Hanrahan JW. Mucus secretion by single tracheal submucosal glands from normal and cystic fibrosis transmembrane conductance regulator knockout mice. *J Physiol* 580: pp. 301–14, 2007.

[499] Zwartz GJ, and Guilmette RA. Effect of flow rate on particle deposition in a replica of a human nasal airway. *Inhal Toxicol* 13: pp. 109–27, 2001.

[500] Tos M, and Mogensen C. Density of mucous glands in the normal adult nasal septum. *Arch Otorhinolaryngol* 214: pp. 125–33, 1976.

[501] Tos M, and Morgensen C. Density of mucous glands in the normal adult nasal turbinates. *Arch Otorhinolaryngol* 215: pp. 101–11, 1977.

[502] Tos M. Distribution of mucus producing elements in the respiratory tract. Differences between upper and lower airway. *Eur J Respir Dis Suppl* 128 (Pt 1): pp. 269–79, 1983.

[503] Tos M, and Mogensen C. Mucus production in the nasal sinuses. *Acta Otolaryngol Suppl* 360: pp. 131–4, 1979.

[504] Bojsen-Moller F. Topography of the nasal glands in rats and some other mammals. *Anat Rec* 150: pp. 11–24, 1964.

[505] Adams DR. Fine structure of the vomeronasal and septal olfactory epithelia and of glandular structures. *Microsc Res Tech* 23: pp. 86–97, 1992.

[506] Bojsen-Moller F. Glandulae nasales anteriores in the human nose. *Ann Otol Rhinol Laryngol* 74: pp. 363–75, 1965.

[507] Pevsner J, Hwang PM, Sklar PB, Venable JC, and Snyder SH. Odorant-binding protein and its mRNA are localized to lateral nasal gland implying a carrier function. *Proc Natl Acad Sci USA* 85: pp. 2383–7, 1988.

[508] Blatt CM, Taylor CR, and Habal MB. Thermal panting in dogs: the lateral nasal gland, a source of water for evaporative cooling. *Science* 177: pp. 804–5, 1972.

[509] St. George JA, Nishio SJ, Cranz DL, and Plopper CG. Carbohydrate cytochemistry of rhesus monkey tracheal submucosal glands. *Anat Rec* 216: pp. 60–7, 1986.

[510] Widdicombe JH. Accumulation of airway mucus in cystic fibrosis. *Pulm Pharmacol* 7: pp. 225–33, 1994.

[511] Basbaum CB, Jany B, and Finkbeiner WE. The serous cell. *Ann Rev Physiol* 52: pp. 97–113, 1990.

[512] Fischer H, Illek B, Sachs L, Finkbeiner WE, and Widdicombe JH. CFTR and calcium-activated chloride channels in primary cultures of human airway gland cells of serous or mucous phenotype. *Am J Physiol* 299: pp. L585–94, 2010.

[513] Basbaum CB. Regulation of airway secretory cells. *Clin Chest Med* 7: pp. 231–7, 1986.

[514] Shimura S, Sasaki T, Sasaki H, and Takishima T. Contractility of isolated single submucosal gland from trachea. *J Appl Physiol* 60: pp. 1237–47, 1986.

[515] Sorokin SP. On the cytology and cytochemistry of the opossum's bronchial glands. *Am J Anat* 117: pp. 311–38, 1965.

[516] Trout L, Gatzy JT, and Ballard ST. Acetylcholine-induced liquid secretion by bronchial epithelium: role of Cl^- and HCO_3^- transport. *Am J Physiol* 275: pp. L1095–9, 1998.

[517] Lee RJ, and Foskett JK. Mechanisms of Ca^{2+}-stimulated fluid secretion by porcine bronchial submucosal gland serous acinar cells. *Am J Physiol* 298: pp. L210–31, 2010.

[518] Lee RJ, Limberis MP, Hennessy MF, Wilson JM, and Foskett JK. Optical imaging of Ca^{2+}-evoked fluid secretion by murine nasal submucosal gland serous acinar cells. *J Physiol* 582: pp. 1099–124, 2007.

[519] Lee RJ, Harlow JM, Limberis MP, Wilson JM, and Foskett JK. HCO_3^- secretion by murine nasal submucosal gland serous acinar cells during Ca^{2+}-stimulated fluid secretion. *J Gen Physiol* 132: pp. 161–83, 2008.

[520] Joo NS, Krouse ME, Wu JV, Saenz Y, Jayaraman S, Verkman AS, and Wine JJ. HCO_3^- transport in relation to mucus secretion from submucosal glands. *JOP* 2: pp. 280–4, 2001.

[521] Joo NS, Wu JV, Krouse ME, Saenz Y, and Wine JJ. Optical method for quantifying rates of mucus secretion from single submucosal glands. *Am J Physiol* 281: pp. L458–68, 2001.

[522] Joo NS, Irokawa T, Wu JV, Robbins RC, Whyte RI, and Wine JJ. Absent secretion to vasoactive intestinal peptide in cystic fibrosis airway glands. *J Biol Chem* 277: pp. 50710–5, 2002.

[523] Choi JY, Khansaheb M, Joo NS, Krouse ME, Robbins RC, Weill D, and Wine JJ. Substance P stimulates human airway submucosal gland secretion mainly via a CFTR-dependent process. *J Clin Invest* 119: pp. 1189–200, 2009.

[524] Choi JY, Joo NS, Krouse ME, Wu JV, Robbins RC, Ianowski JP, Hanrahan JW, and Wine JJ. Synergistic airway gland mucus secretion in response to vasoactive intestinal peptide and carbachol is lost in cystic fibrosis. *J Clin Invest* 117: pp. 3118–27, 2007.

[525] Quinton PM. Composition and control of secretions from tracheal bronchial submucosal glands. *Nature* 279: pp. 551–2, 1979.

[526] Jayaraman S, Joo NS, Reitz B, Wine JJ, and Verkman AS. Submucosal gland secretions in airways from cystic fibrosis patients have normal [Na$^+$] and pH but elevated viscosity. *Proc Natl Acad Sci USA* 98: pp. 8119–23, 2001.

[527] Partanen M, Laitinen A, Hervonen A, Toivanen M, and Laitinen LA. Catecholamine- and acetylcholinesterase-containing nerves in human lower respiratory tract. *Histochemistry* 76: pp. 175–88, 1982.

[528] Pack RJ, and Richardson PS. The aminergic innervation of the human bronchus: A light and electron microscopic study. *J Anat* 138: pp. 493–502, 1984.

[529] Murlas C, Nadel JA, and Basbaum CB. A morphometric analysis of the autonomic innervation of cat tracheal glands. *J Auton Nerv Syst* 2: pp. 233–7, 1980.

[530] Laitinen A, Partanen M, Hervonen A, Pelto-Huikko M, and Laitinen LA. VIP like immunoreactive nerves in human respiratory tract. Light and electron microscopic study. *Histochemistry* 82: pp. 313–9, 1985.

[531] Baraniuk JN, and Kaliner M. Neuropeptides and nasal secretion. *Am J Physiol* 261: pp. L223–35, 1991.

[532] Shimura S, and Takishima T. Airway submucosal gland secretion. In: *Airway Secretion. Physiological Bases for the Control of Mucous Hypersecretion*, edited by Shimura S and Takishima T. New York: Marcel Dekker, Inc., 1994, pp. 325–98.

[533] Florey H, Carleton HM, and Wells AQ. Mucus secretion in the trachea. *Br J Exp Pathol* 13: pp. 269–84, 1932.

[534] Baker B, Peatfield AC, and Richardson PS. Nervous control of mucin secretion into human bronchi. *J Physiol* 365: pp. 297–305, 1985.

[535] Phipps RJ, Richardson PS, Pack RJ, and Wright N. Sympathomimetic drugs stimulate the output of secretory glycoproteins from human bronchi *in vitro*. *Clin Sci* 63: pp. 23–8, 1982.

[536] Peatfield AC, Barnes PJ, Bratcher C, Nadel JA, and Davis B. Vasoactive intestinal peptide stimulates tracheal submucosal gland secretion in ferret. *Am Rev Respir Dis* 128: pp. 89–93, 1983.

[537] Shimura S, Sasaki T, Ikeda K, Sasaki H, and Takishima T. VIP augments cholinergic-induced glycoconjugate secretion in tracheal submucosal glands. *J Appl Physiol* 65: pp. 2537–44, 1988.

[538] Khansaheb M, Choi JY, Joo NS, Yang YM, Krouse M, and Wine JJ. Properties of substance P-stimulated mucus secretion from porcine tracheal submucosal glands. *Am J Physiol* 300: pp. L370–9, 2011.

[539] Barnes PJ, and Basbaum CB. Mapping of adrenergic receptors in the trachea by autoradiography. *Exp Lung Res* 5: pp. 183–92, 1983.

[540] Peatfield AC, and Richardson PS. The control of mucin secretion into the lumen of the cat

trachea by α- and β-adrenoceptors, and their relative involvement during sympathetic nerve stimulation. *Eur J Pharmacol* 81: pp. 617–26, 1982.

[541]   Phipps RJ, Nadel JA, and Davis B. Effect of alpha-adrenergic stimulation on mucus secretion and on ion transport in cat trachea in vitro. *Am Rev Respir Dis* 121: pp. 359–65, 1980.

[542]   Gallagher JT, Hall RL, Phipps RJ, Jeffery PK, Kent PW, and Richardson PS. Mucus-glycoproteins (mucins) of the cat trachea: characterisation and control of secretion. *Biochim Biophys Acta* 886: pp. 243–54, 1986.

[543]   Ueki I, and Nadel JA. Differences in total protein concentration in submucosal gland fluid: α-adrenergic vs cholinergic. *Fed Proc* 40: pp. 622, 1981.

[544]   Leikauf GD, Ueki IF, and Nadel JA. Autonomic regulation of viscoelasticity of cat tracheal gland secretions. *J Appl Physiol* 56: pp. 426–30, 1984.

[545]   Martens CJ, Inglis SK, Valentine VG, Garrison J, Conner GE, and Ballard ST. Mucous solids and liquid secretion by airways: studies with normal pig, cystic fibrosis human, and non-cystic fibrosis human bronchi. *Am J Physiol* 301: pp. L236–46, 2011.

[546]   Fahy JV, and Dickey BF. Airway mucus function and dysfunction. *N Engl J Med* 363: pp. 2233–47, 2010.

[547]   Aoshiba K, and Nagai A. Differences in airway remodeling between asthma and chronic obstructive pulmonary disease. *Clin Rev Allergy Immunol* 27: pp. 35–43, 2004.

[548]   Chung KF, and Adcock IM. Multifaceted mechanisms in COPD: inflammation, immunity, and tissue repair and destruction. *Eur Resp J* 31: pp. 1334–56, 2008.

[549]   Mall MA. Role of cilia, mucus, and airway surface liquid in mucociliary dysfunction: lessons from mouse models. *J Aerosol Med Pulm Drug Deliv* 21: pp. 13–24, 2008.

[550]   Jeffery PK. Remodeling and inflammation of bronchi in asthma and chronic obstructive pulmonary disease. *Proc Am Thorac Soc* 1: pp. 176–83, 2004.

[551]   Downey DG, Bell SC, and Elborn JS. Neutrophils in cystic fibrosis. *Thorax* 64: pp. 81–8, 2009.

[552]   Chung KF. Inflammatory mediators in chronic obstructive pulmonary disease. *Curr Drug Targets Inflamm Allergy* 4: pp. 619–25, 2005.

[553]   Machen TE. Innate immune response in CF airway epithelia: hyperinflammatory? *Am J Physiol* 291: pp. C218–30, 2006.

[554]   Holgate ST. The sentinel role of the airway epithelium in asthma pathogenesis. *Immunol Rev* 242: pp. 205–19, 2011.

[555]   Quinton PM. Role of epithelial HCO_3^- transport in mucin secretion: lessons from cystic fibrosis. *Am J Physiol* 299: pp. C1222–33, 2010.

[556]   Hays SR, and Fahy JV. Characterizing mucous cell remodeling in cystic fibrosis: relationship to neutrophils. *Am J Respir Crit Care Med* 174: pp. 1018–24, 2006.

[557] Restrepo GL, and Heard BE. Mucous gland enlargement in chronic bronchitis: extent of enlargement in the tracheo-bronchial tree. *Thorax* 18: pp. 334–9, 1963.

[558] Reid L. Measurement of the bronchial mucous gland layer: a diagnostic yardstick in chronic bronchitis. *Thorax* 15: pp. 132–41, 1960.

[559] Thurlbeck WM, and Angus GE. A distribution curve for chronic bronchitis. *Thorax* 19: pp. 436–42, 1964.

[560] Dunnill MS, Massarella GR, and Anderson JA. A comparison of the quantitative anatomy of the bronchi in normal subjects, in status asthmaticus, in chronic bronchitis, and in emphysema. *Thorax* 24: pp. 176–9, 1969.

[561] Dunnill MS. The pathology of asthma, with special reference to changes in the bronchial mucosa. *J Clin Path* 13: pp. 27–33, 1960.

[562] Oberholzer M, Dalquen P, Wyss M, and Rohr HP. The applicability of the gland/wall ratio (Reid-Index) to clinicopathological correlation studies. *Thorax* 33: pp. 779–84, 1978.

[563] Aikawa T, Shimura S, Sasaki H, Takishima T, Yaegashi H, and Takahashi T. Morphometric analysis of intraluminal mucus in airways in chronic obstructive pulmonary disease. *Am Rev Respir Dis* 140: pp. 477–82, 1989.

[564] Ciba Guest Symposium. Terminology, definitions and classifications of chronic pulmonary emphysema and related conditions. *Thorax* 14: pp. 286–99, 1959.

[565] Lapperre TS, Sont JK, van Schadewijk A, Gosman MM, Postma DS, Bajema IM, Timens W, Mauad T, and Hiemstra PS. Smoking cessation and bronchial epithelial remodelling in COPD: a cross-sectional study. *Respir Res* 8: p. 85, 2007.

[566] Mullen JB, Wright JL, Wiggs BR, Pare PD, and Hogg JC. Structure of central airways in current smokers and ex-smokers with and without mucus hypersecretion: relationship to lung function. *Thorax* 42: pp. 843–8, 1987.

[567] Cosio M, Ghezzo H, Hogg JC, Corbin R, Loveland M, Dosman J, and Macklem PT. The relations between structural changes in small airways and pulmonary-function tests. *N Engl J Med* 298: pp. 1277–81, 1978.

[568] Araya J, Cambier S, Markovics JA, Wolters P, Jablons D, Hill A, Finkbeiner W, Jones K, Broaddus VC, Sheppard D, Barzcak A, Xiao Y, Erle DJ, and Nishimura SL. Squamous metaplasia amplifies pathologic epithelial–mesenchymal interactions in COPD patients. *J Clin Invest* 117: pp. 3551–62, 2007.

[569] Takizawa H, Tanaka M, Takami K, Ohtoshi T, Ito K, Satoh M, Okada Y, Yamasawa F, Nakahara K, and Umeda A. Increased expression of transforming growth factor-beta1 in small airway epithelium from tobacco smokers and patients with chronic obstructive pulmonary disease (COPD). *Am J Respir Crit Care Med* 163: pp. 1476–83, 2001.

[570] Tos M, and Moller K. Goblet-cell density in human bronchus in chronic bronchitis. *Arch Otolaryngol* 109: pp. 673–6, 1983.

[571]   Innes AL, Woodruff PG, Ferrando RE, Donnelly S, Dolganov GM, Lazarus SC, and Fahy JV. Epithelial mucin stores are increased in the large airways of smokers with airflow obstruction. *Chest* 130: pp. 1102–8, 2006.

[572]   O'Donnell RA, Richter A, Ward J, Angco G, Mehta A, Rousseau K, Swallow DM, Holgate ST, Djukanovic R, Davies DE, and Wilson SJ. Expression of ErbB receptors and mucins in the airways of long term current smokers. *Thorax* 59: pp. 1032–40, 2004.

[573]   Trevisani L, Sartori S, Bovolenta MR, Mazzoni M, Pazzi P, Putinati S, and Potena A. Structural characterization of the bronchial epithelium of subjects with chronic bronchitis and in asymptomatic smokers. *Respiration* 59: pp. 136–44, 1992.

[574]   Saetta M, Turato G, Baraldo S, Zanin A, Braccioni F, Mapp CE, Maestrelli P, Cavallesco G, Papi A, and Fabbri LM. Goblet cell hyperplasia and epithelial inflammation in peripheral airways of smokers with both symptoms of chronic bronchitis and chronic airflow limitation. *Am J Respir Crit Care Med* 161: pp. 1016–21, 2000.

[575]   Caramori G, Di Gregorio C, Carlstedt I, Guzzinati I, Adcock IM, Barnes PJ, Ciaccia A, Cavellesco G, Chung KF, and Papi A. Mucin expression in peripheral airways of patients with chronic obstructive pulmonary disease. *Histopathology* 45: pp. 477–84, 2004.

[576]   Thurlbeck WM. *Chronic Airflow Obstruction in Lung Disease*. Philadelphia: W. B. Saunders, 1976.

[577]   De Haller R, and Reid L. Adult chronic bronchitis: morphology, histochemistry and vascularization of the bronchial mucous glands. *Med Thorac* 22: pp. 549–67, 1965.

[578]   Douglas AN. Quantitative study of bronchial mucous gland enlargement. *Thorax* 35: pp. 198–201, 1980.

[579]   Takizawa T, and Thurlbeck WM. A comparative study of four methods of assessing the morphologic changes in chronic bronchitis. *Am Rev Respir Dis* 103: pp. 774–83, 1971.

[580]   Kirkham S, Sheehan JK, Knight D, Richardson PS, and Thornton DJ. Heterogeneity of airways mucus: variations in the amounts and glycoforms of the major oligomeric mucins MUC5AC and MUC5B. *Biochem J* 361: pp. 537–46, 2002.

[581]   Kirkham S, Kolsum U, Rousseau K, Singh D, Vestbo J, and Thornton DJ. MUC5B is the major mucin in the gel phase of sputum in chronic obstructive pulmonary disease. *Am J Respir Crit Care Med* 178: pp. 1033–9, 2008.

[582]   Mullen JB, Wright JL, Wiggs BR, Pare PD, and Hogg JC. Reassessment of inflammation of airways in chronic bronchitis. *Br Med J (Clin Res Ed)* 291: pp. 1235–9, 1985.

[583]   Pesci A, Rossi GA, Bertorelli G, Aufiero A, Zanon P, and Olivieri D. Mast cells in the airway lumen and bronchial mucosa of patients with chronic bronchitis. *Am J Respir Crit Care Med* 149: pp. 1311–6, 1994.

[584]   Zhu J, Qiu Y, Valobra M, Qiu S, Majumdar S, Matin D, De Rose V, and Jeffery PK. Plasma

cells and IL-4 in chronic bronchitis and chronic obstructive pulmonary disease. *Am J Respir Crit Care Med* 175: pp. 1125–33, 2007.

[585] Saetta M, Turato G, Facchini FM, Corbino L, Lucchini RE, Casoni G, Maestrelli P, Mapp CE, Ciaccia A, and Fabbri LM. Inflammatory cells in the bronchial glands of smokers with chronic bronchitis. *Am J Respir Crit Care Med* 156: pp. 1633–9, 1997.

[586] Gross NJ, Co E, and Skorodin MS. Cholinergic bronchomotor tone in COPD. Estimates of its amount in comparison with that in normal subjects. *Chest* 96: pp. 984–7, 1989.

[587] Lucchini RE, Facchini F, Turato G, Saetta M, Caramori G, Ciaccia A, Maestrelli P, Springall DR, Polak JM, Fabbri L, and Mapp CE. Increased VIP-positive nerve fibers in the mucous glands of subjects with chronic bronchitis. *Am J Respir Crit Care Med* 156: pp. 1963–8, 1997.

[588] Kuyper LM, Pare PD, Hogg JC, Lambert RK, Ionescu D, Woods R, and Bai TR. Characterization of airway plugging in fatal asthma. *Am J Med* 115: pp. 6–11, 2003.

[589] Carroll NG, Mutavdzic S, and James AL. Distribution and degranulation of airway mast cells in normal and asthmatic subjects. *Eur Respir J* 19: pp. 879–85, 2002.

[590] Green FH, Williams DJ, James A, McPhee LJ, Mitchell I, and Maud T. Increased myoepithelial cells of bronchial submucosal glands in fatal asthma. *Thorax* 65: pp. 32–8, 2010.

[591] Shimura S, Andoh Y, Haraguchi M, and Shirato K. Continuity of airway goblet cells and intraluminal mucus in the airways of patients with bronchial asthma. *Eur Respir J* 9: 1395–401, 1996.

[592] Aikawa T, Shimura S, Sasaki H, Ebina M, and Takishima T. Marked goblet cell hyperplasia with mucus accumulation in the airways of patients who died of severe acute asthma attack. *Chest* 101: 916–21, 1992.

[593] Sheehan JK, Howard M, Richardson PS, Longwill T, and Thornton DJ. Physical characterization of a low-charge glycoform of the MUC5B mucin comprising the gel-phase of an asthmatic respiratory mucous plug. *Biochem J* 338: 507–13, 1999.

[594] Carroll N, Elliot J, Morton A, and James A. The structure of large and small airways in nonfatal and fatal asthma. *Am Rev Respir Dis* 147: pp. 405–10, 1993.

[595] Takizawa T, and Thurlbeck W. Muscle and mucous gland size in the major bronchi of patients with chronic bronchitis, asthma, and asthmatic bronchitis. *Am Rev Respir Dis* 104: pp. 331–6, 1971.

[596] Ordonez CL, Khashayar R, Wong HH, Ferrando R, Wu R, Hyde DM, Hotchkiss JA, Zhang Y, Novikov A, Dolganov G, and Fahy JV. Mild and moderate asthma is associated with airway goblet cell hyperplasia and abnormalities in mucin gene expression. *Am J Respir Crit Care Med* 163: pp. 517–23, 2001.

[597] Agrawal A, Rengarajan S, Adler KB, Ram A, Ghosh B, Fahim M, and Dickey BF. Inhibition

of mucin secretion with MARCKS-related peptide improves airway obstruction in a mouse model of asthma. *J Appl Physiol* 102: pp. 399–405, 2007.

[598] Montefort S, Roberts JA, Beasley R, Holgate ST, and Roche WR. The site of disruption of the bronchial epithelium in asthmatic and non-asthmatic subjects. *Thorax* 47: pp. 499–503, 1992.

[599] Laitinen LA, Heino M, Laitinen A, Kava T, and Haahtela T. Damage of the airway epithelium and bronchial reactivity in patients with asthma. *Am Rev Respir Dis* 131: pp. 599–606, 1985.

[600] Naylor B. The shedding of the mucosa of the bronchial tree in asthma. *Thorax* 17: pp. 69–72, 1962.

[601] Wardlaw AJ, Dunnette S, Gleich GJ, Collins JV, and Kay AB. Eosinophils and mast cells in bronchoalveolar lavage in subjects with mild asthma. Relationship to bronchial hyperreactivity. *Am Rev Respir Dis* 137: pp. 62–9, 1988.

[602] Beasley R, Roche WR, Roberts JA, and Holgate ST. Cellular events in the bronchi in mild asthma and after bronchial provocation. *Am Rev Respir Dis* 139: pp. 806–17, 1989.

[603] Ordonez C, Ferrando R, Hyde DM, Wong HH, and Fahy JV. Epithelial desquamation in asthma: artifact or pathology? *Am J Respir Crit Care Med* 162: pp. 2324–9, 2000.

[604] Chung NC, Illek B, Widdicombe JH, and Fischer H. Measurement of nasal potential difference in mild asthmatics. *Chest* 123: pp. 1467–71, 2003.

[605] Ilowite JS, Bennett WD, Sheetz MS, Groth ML, and Nierman DM. Permeability of the bronchial mucosa to ^{99}mTc-DTPA in asthma. *Am Rev Respir Dis* 139: pp. 1139–43, 1989.

[606] Brogan TD, Ryley HC, Neal L, and Yassa J. Soluble proteins of bronchopulmonary secretions from patients with cystic fibrosis, asthma, and bronchitis. *Thorax* 30: pp. 72–9, 1975.

[607] Innes AL, Carrington SD, Thornton DJ, Kirkham S, Rousseau K, Dougherty RH, Raymond WW, Caughey GH, Muller SJ, and Fahy JV. Ex vivo sputum analysis reveals impairment of protease-dependent mucus degradation by plasma proteins in acute asthma. *Am J Respir Crit Care Med* 180: pp. 203–10, 2009.

[608] Ribeiro CM, Paradiso AM, Schwab U, Perez-Vilar J, Jones L, O'Neal W, and Boucher RC. Chronic airway infection/inflammation induces a Ca^{2+}i-dependent hyperinflammatory response in human cystic fibrosis airway epithelia. *J Biol Chem* 280: pp. 17798–806, 2005.

[609] Lopez-Souza N, Dolganov G, Dubin R, Sachs LA, Sassina L, Sporer H, Yagi S, Schnurr D, Boushey HA, and Widdicombe JH. Resistance of differentiated human airway epithelium to infection by rhinovirus. *Am J Physiol* 286: pp. L373–81, 2004.

[610] Whitcutt MJ, Adler KB, and Wu R. A biphasic chamber system for maintaining polarity of differentiation of cultured respiratory tract epithelial cells. *In Vitro* 24: pp. 420–8, 1988.

[611] Widdicombe JH, Sachs LA, and Finkbeiner WE. Effects of growth surface on differentiation of cultures of human tracheal epithelium. *In Vitro* 39A: pp. 51–5, 2003.

[612] Widdicombe JH, Sachs LA, Morrow JL, and Finkbeiner WE. Expansion of cultures of human tracheal epithelium with maintenance of differentiated structure and function. *Biotechniques* 39: pp. 249–55, 2005.

[613] Finkbeiner WE, and Widdicombe JH. Serial propagation of cells from human tracheobronchial glands. *In Vitro* 30A: pp. 817–8, 1994.

[614] Zabner J, Karp P, Seiler M, Phillips SL, Mitchell CJ, Saavedra M, Welsh M, and Klingelhutz AJ. Development of cystic fibrosis and noncystic fibrosis airway cell lines. *Am J Physiol* 284: L844–54, 2003.

[615] Sachs LA, Finkbeiner WE, and Widdicombe JH. Effects of media on differentiation of cultured human tracheal epithelium. *In Vitro* 39A: pp. 56–62, 2003.

[616] Bucchieri F, Puddicombe SM, Lordan JL, Richter A, Buchanan D, Wilson SJ, Ward J, Zummo G, Howarth PH, Djukanovic R, Holgate ST, and Davies DE. Asthmatic bronchial epithelium is more susceptible to oxidant-induced apoptosis. *Am J Respir Cell Mol Biol* 27: pp. 179–85, 2002.

[617] Wark PA, Johnston SL, Bucchieri F, Powell R, Puddicombe S, Laza-Stanca V, Holgate ST, and Davies DE. Asthmatic bronchial epithelial cells have a deficient innate immune response to infection with rhinovirus. *J Exp Med* 201: pp. 937–47, 2005.

[618] Puddicombe SM, Torres-Lozano C, Richter A, Bucchieri F, Lordan JL, Howarth PH, Vrugt B, Albers R, Djukanovic R, Holgate ST, Wilson SJ, and Davies DE. Increased expression of p21(waf) cyclin-dependent kinase inhibitor in asthmatic bronchial epithelium. *Am J Respir Cell Mol Biol* 28: pp. 61–8, 2003.

[619] Lordan JL, Bucchieri F, Richter A, Konstantinidis A, Holloway JW, Thornber M, Puddicombe SM, Buchanan D, Wilson SJ, Djukanovic R, Holgate ST, and Davies DE. Cooperative effects of Th2 cytokines and allergen on normal and asthmatic bronchial epithelial cells. *J Immunol* 169: pp. 407–14, 2002.

[620] Xiao C, Puddicombe SM, Field S, Haywood J, Broughton-Head V, Puxeddu I, Haitchi HM, Vernon-Wilson E, Sammut D, Bedke N, Cremin C, Sones J, Djukanovic R, Howarth PH, Collins JE, Holgate ST, Monk P, and Davies DE. Defective epithelial barrier function in asthma. *J Allergy Clin Immunol* 128: pp. 549–56, 2011.

[621] Parker J, Sarlang S, Thavagnanam S, Williamson G, O'Donoghue D, Villenave R, Power U, Shields M, Heaney L, and Skibinski G. A 3-D well-differentiated model of pediatric bronchial epithelium demonstrates unstimulated morphological differences between asthmatic and nonasthmatic cells. *Pediatr Res* 67: pp. 17–22, 2010.

[622] Bayram H, Devalia JL, Khair OA, Abdelaziz MM, Sapsford RJ, Sagai M, and Davies RJ. Comparison of ciliary activity and inflammatory mediator release from bronchial epithelial cells of nonatopic nonasthmatic subjects and atopic asthmatic patients and the effect of diesel exhaust particles in vitro. *J Allergy Clin Immunol* 102: pp. 771–82, 1998.

[623] Bayram H, Devalia JL, Sapsford RJ, Ohtoshi T, Miyabara Y, Sagai M, and Davies RJ. The effect of diesel exhaust particles on cell function and release of inflammatory mediators from human bronchial epithelial cells in vitro. *Am J Respir Cell Mol Biol* 18: pp. 441–8, 1998.

[624] Bayram H, Sapsford RJ, Abdelaziz MM, and Khair OA. Effect of ozone and nitrogen dioxide on the release of proinflammatory mediators from bronchial epithelial cells of nonatopic nonasthmatic subjects and atopic asthmatic patients in vitro. *J Allergy Clin Immunol* 107: pp. 287–94, 2001.

[625] Gras D, Bourdin A, Vachier I, de Senneville L, Bonnans C, and Chanez P. An ex vivo model of severe asthma using reconstituted human bronchial epithelium. *J Allergy Clin Immunol* 129: pp. 1259–66, 2012.

[626] Kicic A, Sutanto EN, Stevens PT, Knight DA, and Stick SM. Intrinsic biochemical and functional differences in bronchial epithelial cells of children with asthma. *Am J Respir Crit Care Med* 174: pp. 1110–8, 2006.

[627] Kicic A, Hallstrand TS, Sutanto EN, Stevens PT, Kobor MS, Taplin C, Pare PD, Beyer RP, Stick SM, and Knight DA. Decreased fibronectin production significantly contributes to dysregulated repair of asthmatic epithelium. *Am J Respir Crit Care Med* 181: pp. 889–98, 2010.

[628] Freishtat RJ, Watson AM, Benton AS, Iqbal SF, Pillai DK, Rose MC, and Hoffman EP. Asthmatic airway epithelium is intrinsically inflammatory and mitotically dyssynchronous. *Am J Respir Cell Mol Biol* 44: pp. 863–9, 2011.

[629] Andersen D. Cystic fibrosis of the pancreas. *J Chron Dis* 7: pp. 58–90, 1958.

[630] Gibson RL, Burns JL, and Ramsey BW. Pathophysiology and management of pulmonary infections in cystic fibrosis. *Am J Respir Crit Care Med* 168: pp. 918–51, 2003.

[631] Moskwa P, Lorentzen D, Excoffon KJDA, Zabner J, McCray PB, Nauseef WM, Dupuy C, and Banfi B. A novel host defense system of airways is defective in cystic fibrosis. *Am J Resp Crit Care Med* 175: pp. 174–83, 2007.

[632] Singh PK, Schaefer AL, Parsek MR, Moninger TO, Welsh MJ, and Greenberg EP. Quorum-sensing signals indicate that cystic fibrosis lungs are infected with bacterial biofilms. *Nature* 407: pp. 762–4, 2000.

[633] Bedrossian CW, Greenberg SD, Singer DB, Hansen JJ, and Rosenberg HS. The lung in cystic fibrosis. A quantitative study including prevalence of pathologic findings among different age groups. *Human Pathol* 7: pp. 195–204, 1976.

[634] Shak S, Capon DJ, Hellmiss R, Marsters SA, and Baker CL. Recombinant human DNase I

reduces the viscosity of cystic fibrosis sputum. *Proc Natl Acad Sci USA* 87: pp. 9188–92, 1990.

[635] Burgel PR, Montani D, Danel C, Dusser DJ, and Nadel JA. A morphometric study of mucins and small airway plugging in cystic fibrosis. *Thorax* 62: pp. 153–61, 2007.

[636] Ostedgaard LS, Meyerholz DK, Chen JH, Pezzulo AA, Karp PH, Rokhlina T, Ernst SE, Hanfland RA, Reznikov LR, Ludwig PS, Rogan MP, Davis GJ, Dohrn CL, Wohlford-Lenane C, Taft PJ, Rector MV, Hornick E, Nassar BS, Samuel M, Zhang Y, Richter SS, Uc A, Shilyansky J, Prather RS, McCray PB, Jr., Zabner J, Welsh MJ, and Stoltz DA. The DeltaF508 mutation causes CFTR misprocessing and cystic fibrosis-like disease in pigs. *Sci Transl Med* 3: p. 74ra24, 2011.

[637] Oppenheimer EH, and Esterly JR. Pathology of cystic fibrosis: review of the literature and comparison with 146 autopsied cases. *Perspect Pediatr Pathol* 2: pp. 241–78, 1975.

[638] Reid L, and de Haller R. The bronchial mucous glands—their hypertrophy and change in intracellular mucus. *Mod Probl Paediat* 10: pp. 195–9, 1967.

[639] Sturgess J, and Imrie J. Quantitative evaluation of the development of tracheal submucosal glands in infants with cystic fibrosis and control infants. *Am J Pathol* 106: pp. 303–11, 1982.

[640] Oppenheimer EH. Similarity of the tracheobronchial mucous glands and epithelium in infants with and without cystic fibrosis. *Human Pathol* 12: pp. 36–48, 1981.

[641] Barthelson RA, and Widdicombe JH. The cyclic adenosine monophosphate-dependent protein kinase in cystic fibrosis tracheal epithelium. *J Clin Invest* 80: pp. 1799–802, 1987.

[642] Pizurki L, Morris MA, Chanson M, Solomon M, Pavirani A, Bouchardy I, and Suter S. Cystic fibrosis transmembrane conductance regulator does not affect neutrophil migration across cystic fibrosis airway epithelial monolayers. *Am J Pathol* 156: pp. 1407–16, 2000.

[643] Poulsen JH, Fischer H, Illek B, and Machen TE. Bicarbonate conductance and pH regulatory capability of cystic fibrosis transmembrane conductance regulator. *Proc Natl Acad Sci* 91: pp. 5340–4, 1994.

[644] McShane D, Davies JC, Davies MG, Bush A, Geddes DM, and Alton EW. Airway surface pH in subjects with cystic fibrosis. *Eur Respir J* 21: pp. 37–42, 2003.

[645] Grubb BR, Paradiso AM, and Boucher RC. Anomalies in ion transport in CF mouse tracheal epithelium. *Am J Physiol* 267: pp. C293–300, 1994.

[646] Cho DY, Hwang PH, Illek B, and Fischer H. Acid and base secretion in freshly excised nasal tissue from cystic fibrosis patients with DeltaF508 mutation. *Int Forum Allergy Rhinol* 1: pp. 123–7, 2011.

[647] Muchekehu RW, and Quinton PM. A new role for bicarbonate secretion in cervico-uterine mucus release. *J Physiol* 588: pp. 2329–42, 2010.

[648] Garcia MA, Yang N, and Quinton PM. Normal mouse intestinal mucus release requires

cystic fibrosis transmembrane regulator-dependent bicarbonate secretion. *J Clin Invest* 119: pp. 2613–22, 2009.

[649]   Salinas D, Haggie PM, Thiagarajah JR, Song Y, Rosbe K, Finkbeiner WE, Nielson DW, and Verkman AS. Submucosal gland dysfunction as a primary defect in cystic fibrosis. *FASEB J* 19: pp. 431–3, 2005.

[650]   Thiagarajah JR, Song Y, Haggie PM, and Verkman AS. A small molecule CFTR inhibitor produces cystic fibrosis-like submucosal gland fluid secretions in normal airways *Faseb J* 18: pp. 875–7, 2004.

[651]   Jiang C, Finkbeiner WE, Widdicombe JH, and Miller SS. Fluid transport across cultures of human tracheal glands is altered in cystic fibrosis. *J Physiol* 501: pp. 637–47, 1997.

[652]   Joo NS, Cho HJ, Khansaheb M, and Wine JJ. Hyposecretion of fluid from tracheal submucosal glands of CFTR-deficient pigs. *J Clin Invest* 120: pp. 3161–6, 2010.

[653]   Haxhiu MA, van Lunteren E, and Cherniack NS. Central effects of tachykinin peptides on tracheal secretion. *Respir Physiol* 86: pp. 405–14, 1991.

[654]   Baniak N, Luan X, Grunow A, Machen TE, and Ianowski JP. The cytokines interleukin-1β and tumor necrosis factor-α stimulate CFTR-mediated fluid secretion by swine airway submucosal glands. *Am J Physiol* 303: pp. L327–33, 2012.

[655]   Gowen CW, Lawson EE, Gingras-Leatherman J, Gatzy JT, Boucher RC, and Knowles MR. Increased nasal potential difference and amiloride sensitivity in neonates with cystic fibrosis. *J Pediatr* 108: pp. 517–21, 1986.

[656]   Stutts MJ, Canessa CM, Olsen JC, Hamrick M, Cohn JA, Rossier BC, and Boucher RC. CFTR as a cAMP-dependent regulator of sodium channels. *Science* 269: pp. 847–50, 1995.

[657]   Nagel G, Barbry P, Chabot H, Brochiero E, Hartung K, and Grygorczyk R. CFTR fails to inhibit the epithelial sodium channel ENaC expressed in *Xenopus laevis* oocytes. *J Physiol* 564: pp. 671–82, 2005.

[658]   Stutts MJ, Knowles MR, Gatzy JT, and Boucher RC. Oxygen consumption and ouabain binding sites in cystic fibrosis nasal epithelium. *Pediatr Res* 20: pp. 1316–20, 1986.

[659]   Rubenstein RC, Lockwood SR, Lide E, Bauer R, Suaud L, and Grumbach Y. Regulation of endogenous ENaC functional expression by CFTR and DeltaF508-CFTR in airway epithelial cells. *Am J Physiol* 300: pp. L88–101, 2011.

[660]   Stutts MJ, Rossier BC, and Boucher RC. Cystic fibrosis transmembrane conductance regulator inverts protein kinase A-mediated regulation of epithelial sodium channel single channel kinetics. *J Biol Chem* 272: pp. 14037–40, 1997.

[661]   Ji HL, Chalfant ML, Jovov B, Lockhart JP, Parker SB, Fuller CM, Stanton BA, and Benos DJ. The cytosolic termini of the beta- and gamma-ENaC subunits are involved in the

functional interactions between cystic fibrosis transmembrane conductance regulator and epithelial sodium channel. *J Biol Chem* 275: pp. 27947–56, 2000.

[662] Gentzsch M, Dang H, Dang Y, Garcia-Caballero A, Suchindran H, Boucher RC, and Stutts MJ. The cystic fibrosis transmembrane conductance regulator impedes proteolytic stimulation of the epithelial Na^+ channel. *J Biol Chem* 285: pp. 32227–32, 2010.

[663] Ismailov II, Berdiev BK, Shlyonsky VG, Fuller CM, Prat AG, Jovov B, Cantiello HF, Ausiello DA, and Benos DJ. Role of actin in regulation of epithelial sodium channels by CFTR. *Am J Physiol* 272: pp. C1077–86, 1997.

[664] Bingle L, Barnes FA, Cross SS, Rassl D, Wallace WA, Campos MA, and Bingle CD. Differential epithelial expression of the putative innate immune molecule SPLUNC1 in cystic fibrosis. *Respir Res* 8: p. 79, 2007.

[665] Itani OA, Chen JH, Karp PH, Ernst S, Keshavjee S, Parekh K, Klesney-Tait J, Zabner J, and Welsh MJ. Human cystic fibrosis airway epithelia have reduced Cl^- conductance but not increased Na^+ conductance. *Proc Natl Acad Sci USA* 108: pp. 10260–5, 2011.

[666] Willumsen NJ, and Boucher RC. Transcellular sodium transport in cultured cystic fibrosis human nasal epithelium. *Am J Physiol* 261: pp. C332–41, 1991.

[667] Horisberger JD. ENaC-CFTR interactions: the role of electrical coupling of ion fluxes explored in an epithelial cell model. *Pflugers Arch* 445: pp. 522–8, 2003.

[668] Duszyk M, and French AS. An analytical model of ionic movements in airway epithelial cells. *J Theor Biol* 151: pp. 231–47, 1991.

[669] Smith JJ, Travis SM, Greenberg EP, and Welsh MJ. Cystic fibrosis airway epithelia fail to kill bacteria because of abnormal airway surface fluid. *Cell* 85: pp. 229–36, 1996.

[670] Travis SM, Conway BA, Zabner J, Smith JJ, Anderson NN, Singh PK, Greenberg EP, and Welsh MJ. Activity of abundant antimicrobials of the human airway. *Am J Respir Cell Mol Biol* 20: pp. 872–9, 1999.

[671] Goldman MJ, Anderson GM, Stolzenberg ED, Kari UP, Zasloff M, and Wilson JM. Human beta-defensin-1 is a salt-sensitive antibiotic in lung that is inactivated in cystic fibrosis. *Cell* 88: pp. 553–60, 1997.

[672] Conner GE, Wijkstrom-Frei C, Randell SH, Fernandez VE, and Salathe M. The lactoperoxidase system links anion transport to host defense in cystic fibrosis. *FEBS Letters* 581: pp. 271–8, 2007.

[673] Lorentzen D, Durairaj L, Pezzulo AA, Nakano Y, Launspach J, Stoltz DA, Zamba G, McCray PB, Jr., Zabner J, Welsh MJ, Nauseef WM, and Banfi B. Concentration of the antibacterial precursor thiocyanate in cystic fibrosis airway secretions. *Free Radic Biol Med* 50: pp. 1144–50, 2011.

[674] van Klaveren RJ, Demedts M, and Nemery B. Cellular glutathione turnover in vitro, with emphasis on type II pneumocytes. *Eur Respir J* 10: pp. 1392–400, 1997.

[675] Kogan I, Ramjeesingh M, Li C, Kidd JF, Wang Y, Leslie EM, Cole SP, and Bear CE. CFTR directly mediates nucleotide-regulated glutathione flux. *EMBO J* 22: pp. 1981–9, 2003.

[676] Roum JH, Buhl R, McElvaney NG, Borok Z, and Crystal RG. Systemic deficiency of glutathione in cystic fibrosis. *J Appl Physiol* 75: pp. 2419–24, 1993.

[677] Hudson VM. Rethinking cystic fibrosis pathology: the critical role of abnormal reduced glutathione (GSH) transport caused by CFTR mutation. *Free Radic Biol Med* 30: pp. 1440–61, 2001.

[678] Reisin IL, Prat AG, Abraham EH, Amara JF, Gregory RJ, Ausiello DA, and Cantiello HF. The cystic fibrosis transmembrane conductance regulator is a dual ATP and chloride channel. *J Biol Chem* 269: pp. 20584–91, 1994.

[679] Cantiello HF, Jackson GR, Jr., Grosman CF, Prat AG, Borkan SC, Wang Y, Reisin IL, O'Riordan CR, and Ausiello DA. Electrodiffusional ATP movement through the cystic fibrosis transmembrane conductance regulator. *Am J Physiol* 274: pp. C799–809, 1998.

[680] Reddy MM, Quinton PM, Haws C, Wine JJ, Grygorczyk R, Tabcharani JA, Hanrahan JW, Gunderson KL, and Kopito RR. Failure of the cystic fibrosis transmembrane conductance regulator to conduct ATP. *Science* 271: pp. 1876–9, 1996.

[681] Li C, Ramjeesingh M, and Bear CE. Purified cystic fibrosis transmembrane conductance regulator (CFTR) does not function as an ATP channel. *J Biol Chem* 271: pp. 11623–6, 1996.

[682] Barasch J, Kiss B, Prince A, Saiman L, Gruenert D, and Al-Awqati Q. Defective acidification of intracellular organelles in cystic fibrosis. *Nature* 352: pp. 70–3, 1991.

[683] Rhim AD, Stoykova L, Glick MC, and Scanlin TF. Terminal glycosylation in cystic fibrosis (CF): a review emphasizing the airway epithelial cell. *Glycoconj J* 18: pp. 649–59, 2001.

[684] Barriere H, Bagdany M, Bossard F, Okiyoneda T, Wojewodka G, Gruenert D, Radzioch D, and Lukacs GL. Revisiting the role of cystic fibrosis transmembrane conductance regulator and counterion permeability in the pH regulation of endocytic organelles. *Mol Biol Cell* 20: pp. 3125–41, 2009.

[685] Haggie PM, and Verkman AS. Defective organellar acidification as a cause of cystic fibrosis lung disease: reexamination of a recurring hypothesis. *Am J Physiol* 296: pp. L859–67, 2009.

[686] Brockhausen I, Vavasseur F, and Yang X. Biosynthesis of mucin type O-glycans: lack of correlation between glycosyltransferase and sulfotransferase activities and CFTR expression. *Glycoconj J* 18: pp. 685–97, 2001.

[687] Leir SH, Parry S, Palmai-Pallag T, Evans J, Morris HR, Dell A, and Harris A. Mucin glyco-sylation and sulphation in airway epithelial cells is not influenced by cystic fibrosis transmem-brane conductance regulator expression. *Am J Respir Cell Mol Biol* 32: pp. 453–61, 2005.

[688] Reid CJ, Burdick MD, Hollingsworth MA, and Harris A. CFTR expression does not influence glycosylation of an epitope-tagged MUC1 mucin in colon carcinoma cell lines. *Glycobiology* 9: pp. 389–98, 1999.

[689] Shori DK, Kariyawasam HH, Knight RA, Hodson ME, Genter T, Hansen J, Koch C, and Kalogeridis A. Sulphation of the salivary mucin MG1 (MUC-5B) is not correlated to the degree of its sialylation and is unaffected by cystic fibrosis. *Pflugers Arch* 443 Suppl 1: pp. S50–4, 2001.

[690] Stutts MJ, Cotton CU, Yankaskas JR, Knowles MR, Gatzy JT, and Boucher RC. Chloride uptake into cultured airway epithelial cells from cystic fibrosis patients and normal indi-viduals. *Proc Natl Acad Sci USA* 82: pp. 6677–81, 1985.

[691] Li M, McCann JD, Liedtke CM, Nairn AC, Greengard P, and Welsh MJ. Cyclic AMP-dependent protein kinase opens chloride channels in normal but not cystic fibrosis airway epithelium. *Nature* 331: pp. 358–60, 1988.

[692] Schoumacher RA, Shoemaker RL, Halm DR, Tallant EA, Wallace RW, and Frizzell RA. Phosphorylation fails to activate chloride channels from cystic fibrosis airway cells. *Nature* 330: pp. 752–4, 1987.

[693] Solc CK, and Wine JJ. Swelling-induced and depolarization-induced Cl⁻ channels in nor-mal and cystic fibrosis epithelial cells. *Am J Physiol* 261: pp. C658–74, 1991.

[694] Kartner N, Hanrahan JW, Jensen TJ, Naismith AL, Sun S, Ackerley CA, Reyes EF, Tsui L-C, Rommens JM, Bear CE, and Riordan JR. Expression of the cystic fibrosis gene in non-epithelial invertebrate cells produces a regulated anion conductance. *Cell* 64: pp. 681–91, 1991.

[695] Tabcharani JA, Chang X-B, Riordan JR, and Hanrahan JW. Phosphorylation-regulated Cl⁻ channel in CHO cells stably expressing the cystic fibrosis gene. *Nature* 352: pp. 628–31, 1991.

[696] Gabriel SE, Clarke LL, Boucher RC, and Stutts MJ. CFTR and outward rectifying chloride channels are distinct proteins with a regulatory relationship. *Nature* 363: pp. 263–6, 1993.

[697] Egan M, Flotte T, Afione S, Solow R, Zeitlin PL, Carter BJ, and Guggino WB. Defective regulation of outwardly rectifying Cl⁻ channels by protein kinase A corrected by insertion of CFTR. *Nature* 358: pp. 581–4, 1992.

[698] Knowles MR, Clarke LL, and Boucher RC. Activation by extracellular nucleotides of chlo-ride secretion in the airway epithelia of patients with cystic fibrosis. *N Engl J Med* 325: pp. 533–8, 1991.

[699] Grubb BR, Vick RN, and Boucher RC. Hyperabsorption of Na$^+$ and raised Ca^{2+} mediated Cl$^-$ secretion in nasal epithelia of CF mice. *Am J Physiol* 266: pp. C1478–83, 1994.

[700] Ousingsawat J, Kongsuphol P, Schreiber R, and Kunzelmann K. CFTR and TMEM16A are separate but functionally related Cl$^-$ channels. *Cell Physiol Biochem* 28: pp. 715–24, 2011.

[701] Kunzelmann K, Allert N, Kubitz R, Breuer WV, Cabantchik ZI, Normann C, Schumann S, Leipziger J, and Greger R. Forskolin and PMA pretreatment of HT29 cells alters their chloride conductance induced by cAMP, Ca^{2+} and hypotonic cell swelling. *Pflugers Arch* 428: pp. 76–83, 1994.

[702] Kunzelmann K. Control of membrane transport by the cystic fibrosis transmembrane conductance regulator (CFTR). In: *The Cystic Fibrosis Transmembrane Conductance Regulator*, edited by Kirk KL and Dawson DC. Georgetown, Texas: Landes Bioscience, 2003.

[703] Schreiber R, Nitschke R, Greger R, and Kunzelmann K. The cystic fibrosis transmembrane conductance regulator activates aquaporin 3 in airway epithelial cells. *J Biol Chem* 274: pp. 11811–6, 1999.

[704] Chanson M, Scerri I, and Suter S. Defective regulation of gap junctional coupling in cystic fibrosis pancreatic duct cells. *J Clin Invest* 103: pp. 1677–84, 1999.

[705] Ahn W, Kim KH, Lee JA, Kim JY, Choi JY, Moe OW, Milgram SL, Muallem S, and Lee MG. Regulatory interaction between the cystic fibrosis transmembrane conductance regulator and HCO$_3^-$ salvage mechanisms in model systems and the mouse pancreatic duct. *J Biol Chem* 276: pp. 17236–43, 2001.

[706] Lee MG, Choi JY, Luo X, Strickland E, Thomas PJ, and Muallem S. Cystic fibrosis transmembrane conductance regulator regulates luminal Cl$^-$/HCO$_3^-$ exchange in mouse submandibular and pancreatic ducts. *J Biol Chem* 274: pp. 14670–7, 1999.

[707] Jovov B, Ismailov II, Berdiev BK, Fuller CM, Sorscher EJ, Dedman JR, Kaetzel MA, and Benos DJ. Interaction between cystic fibrosis transmembrane conductance regulator and outwardly rectified chloride channels. *J Biol Chem* 270: pp. 29194–200, 1995.

[708] Kunzelmann K. CFTR: interacting with everything? *News Physiol Sci* 16: pp. 167–70, 2001.

[709] Li C, and Naren AP. CFTR chloride channel in the apical compartments: spatiotemporal coupling to its interacting partners. *Integr Biol (Camb)* 2: pp. 161–77, 2010.

[710] Mickle JE, Macek M, Jr., Fulmer-Smentek SB, Egan MM, Schwiebert E, Guggino W, Moss R, and Cutting GR. A mutation in the cystic fibrosis transmembrane conductance regulator gene associated with elevated sweat chloride concentrations in the absence of cystic fibrosis. *Hum Mol Genet* 7: pp. 729–35, 1998.

[711] Tirouvanziam R, de Bentzmann S, Hubeau C, Hinnrasky J, Jacquot J, Peault B, and Puchelle E. Inflammation and infection in naive human cystic fibrosis airway grafts. *Am J Respir Cell Mol Biol* 23: pp. 121–7, 2000.

[712] Estell K, Braunstein G, Tucker T, Varga K, Collawn JF, and Schwiebert LM. Plasma membrane CFTR regulates RANTES expression via its C-terminal PDZ-interacting motif. *Mol Cell Biol* 23: pp. 594–606, 2003.

[713] Winder WW, and Hardie DG. AMP-activated protein kinase, a metabolic master switch: possible roles in type 2 diabetes. *Am J Physiol* 277: pp. E1–10, 1999.

[714] Hallows KR, Raghuram V, Kemp BE, Witters LA, and Foskett JK. Inhibition of cystic fibrosis transmembrane conductance regulator by novel interaction with the metabolic sensor AMP-activated protein kinase. *J Clin Invest* 105: pp. 1711–21, 2000.

[715] King JD, Jr., Fitch AC, Lee JK, McCane JE, Mak DO, Foskett JK, and Hallows KR. AMP-activated protein kinase phosphorylation of the R domain inhibits PKA stimulation of CFTR. *Am J Physiol* 297: pp. C94–101, 2009.

[716] Hallows KR, Fitch AC, Richardson CA, Reynolds PR, Clancy JP, Dagher PC, Witters LA, Kolls JK, and Pilewski JM. Up-regulation of AMP-activated kinase by dysfunctional cystic fibrosis transmembrane conductance regulator in cystic fibrosis airway epithelial cells mitigates excessive inflammation. *J Biol Chem* 281: pp. 4231–41, 2006.

[717] Myerburg MM, King JD, Jr., Oyster NM, Fitch AC, Magill A, Baty CJ, Watkins SC, Kolls JK, Pilewski JM, and Hallows KR. AMPK agonists ameliorate sodium and fluid transport and inflammation in cystic fibrosis airway epithelial cells. *Am J Respir Cell Mol Biol* 42: pp. 676–84, 2010.

[718] Treharne KJ, Xu Z, Chen JH, Best OG, Cassidy DM, Gruenert DC, Hegyi P, Gray MA, Sheppard DN, Kunzelmann K, and Mehta A. Inhibition of protein kinase CK2 closes the CFTR Cl⁻ channel, but has no effect on the cystic fibrosis mutant deltaF508-CFTR. *Cell Physiol Biochem* 24: pp. 347–60, 2009.

[719] Fuller CM, and Benos DJ. CFTR! *Am J Physiol* 263: pp. C267–86, 1992.

[720] Worlitzsch D, Tarran R, Ulrich M, Schwab U, Cekici A, Meyer KC, Birrer P, Bellon G, Berger J, Weiss T, Botzenhart K, Yankaskas JR, Randell S, Boucher RC, and Doring G. Effects of reduced mucus oxygen concentration in airway Pseudomonas infections of cystic fibrosis patients. *J Clin Invest* 109: pp. 317–25, 2002.

[721] Chandel NS, McClintock DS, Feliciano CE, Wood TM, Melendez JA, Rodriguez AM, and Schumacker PT. Reactive oxygen species generated at mitochondrial complex III stabilize hypoxia-inducible factor-1alpha during hypoxia: a mechanism of O2 sensing. *J Biol Chem* 275: pp. 25130–8, 2000.

[722]   Kabe Y, Ando K, Hirao S, Yoshida M, and Handa H. Redox regulation of NF-kappaB activation: distinct redox regulation between the cytoplasm and the nucleus. *Antioxid Redox Signal* 7: pp. 395–403, 2005.

[723]   Kim SK, Woodcroft KJ, Oh SJ, Abdelmegeed MA, and Novak RF. Role of mechanical and redox stress in activation of mitogen-activated protein kinases in primary cultured rat hepatocytes. *Biochem Pharmacol* 70: pp. 1785–95, 2005.

[724]   Ribeiro CM, and Boucher RC. Role of endoplasmic reticulum stress in cystic fibrosis-related airway inflammatory responses. *Proc Am Thorac Soc* 7: pp. 387–94, 2010.

[725]   Ehring GR, Kerschbaum HH, Eder C, Neben AL, Fanger CM, Khoury RM, Negulescu PA, and Cahalan MD. A nongenomic mechanism for progesterone-mediated immunosuppression: inhibition of K^+ channels, Ca^{2+} signaling, and gene expression in T lymphocytes. *J Exp Med* 188: pp. 1593–602, 1998.

[726]   Gruenert DC, Finkbeiner WE, and Widdicombe JH. Culture and transformation of human airway epithelial cells. *Am J Physiol* 268: pp. L347–60, 1995.

[727]   Chanson M, Berclaz PY, Scerri I, Dudez T, Wernke-Dollries K, Pizurki L, Pavirani A, Fiedler MA, and Suter S. Regulation of gap junctional communication by a pro-inflammatory cytokine in cystic fibrosis transmembrane conductance regulator-expressing but not cystic fibrosis airway cells. *Am J Pathol* 158: pp. 1775–84, 2001.

[728]   Sheppard DN, Carson MR, Ostedgaard LS, Denning GM, and Welsh MJ. Expression of cystic fibrosis transmembrane conductance regulator in a model epithelium. *Am J Physiol* 266: pp. L405–13, 1994.

[729]   Perez A, Risma KA, Eckman EA, and Davis PB. Overexpression of R domain eliminates cAMP-stimulated Cl^- secretion in 9/HTEo- cells in culture. *Am J Physiol* 271: pp. L85–92, 1996.

[730]   Shen BQ, Finkbeiner WE, Wine JJ, Mrsny RJ, and Widdicombe JH. Calu-3: a human airway epithelial cell line that shows cAMP-dependent Cl^- secretion. *Am J Physiol* 266: pp. L493–501, 1994.

[731]   Haws C, Finkbeiner WE, Widdicombe JH, and Wine JJ. CFTR in Calu-3 human airway cells: channel properties and role in cAMP-activated Cl^- conductance. *Am J Physiol* 266: pp. L502–12, 1994.

[732]   Palmer ML, Lee SY, Maniak PJ, Carlson D, Fahrenkrug SC, and O'Grady SM. Protease-activated receptor regulation of Cl^- secretion in Calu-3 cells requires prostaglandin release and CFTR activation. *Am J Physiol* 290: pp. C1189–98, 2006.

[733]   Aldallal N, McNaughton EE, Manzel LJ, Richards AM, Zabner J, Ferkol TW, and Look DC. Inflammatory response in airway epithelial cells isolated from patients with cystic fibrosis. *Am J Respir Crit Care Med* 166: pp. 1248–56, 2002.

[734] Jefferson DM, Valentich JD, Marini FC, Grubman SA, Iannuzzi MC, Dorkin HL, Li M, Klinger KW, and Welsh MJ. Expression of normal and cystic fibrosis phenotypes by continuous airway epithelial cell lines. *Am J Physiol* 259: pp. L496–505, 1990.

[735] Becker MN, Sauer MS, Muhlebach MS, Hirsh AJ, Wu Q, Verghese MW, and Randell SH. Cytokine secretion by cystic fibrosis airway epithelial cells. *Am J Respir Crit Care Med* 169: pp. 645–53, 2004.

[736] Wiszniewski L, Jornot L, Dudez T, Pagano A, Rochat T, Lacroix JS, Suter S, and Chanson M. Long-term cultures of polarized airway epithelial cells from patients with cystic fibrosis. *Am J Respir Cell Mol Biol* 34: pp. 39–48, 2006.

[737] Kieninger E, Vareille M, Kopf BS, Blank F, Alves MP, Gisler FM, Latzin P, Casaulta C, Geiser T, Johnston SL, Edwards MR, and Regamey N. Lack of an exaggerated inflammatory response on virus infection in cystic fibrosis. *Eur Respir J* 39: pp. 297–304, 2012.

[738] Perez A, Issler AC, Cotton CU, Kelley TJ, Verkman AS, and Davis PB. CFTR inhibition mimics the cystic fibrosis inflammatory profile. *Am J Physiol* 292: pp. L383–95, 2007.

[739] Saiman L, Cacalano G, Gruenert D, and Prince A. Comparison of adherence of *Pseudomonas aeruginosa* to respiratory epithelial cells from cystic fibrosis patients and healthy subjects. *Infect Immunol* 60: pp. 2808–14, 1992.

[740] Saiman L, and Prince A. Pseudomonas aeruginosa pili bind to asialoGM1 which is increased on the surface of cystic fibrosis epithelial cells. *J Clin Invest* 92: pp. 1875–80, 1993.

[741] Imundo L, Barasch J, Prince A, and Al-Awqati Q. Cystic fibrosis epithelial cells have a receptor for pathogenic bacteria on their apical surface. *Proc Natl Acad Sci USA* 92: pp. 3019–23, 1995.

[742] Bryan R, Kube D, Perez A, Davis P, and Prince A. Overproduction of the CFTR R domain leads to increased levels of asialoGM1 and increased *Pseudomonas aeruginosa* binding by epithelial cells. *Am J Respir Cell Mol Biol* 19: pp. 269–77, 1998.

[743] Hybiske K, Fu Z, Schwarzer C, Tseng J, Do J, Huang N, and Machen TE. Effects of cystic fibrosis transmembrane conductance regulator and DeltaF508CFTR on inflammatory response, ER stress, and Ca^{2+} of airway epithelia. *Am J Physiol* 293: pp. L1250–60, 2007.

[744] Darling KE, Dewar A, and Evans TJ. Role of the cystic fibrosis transmembrane conductance regulator in internalization of *Pseudomonas aeruginosa* by polarized respiratory epithelial cells. *Cell Microbiol* 6: pp. 521–33, 2004.

[745] Schroeder TH, Zaidi T, and Pier GB. Lack of adherence of clinical isolates of *Pseudomonas aeruginosa* to asialo-GM(1) on epithelial cells. *Infect Immun* 69: pp. 719–29, 2001.

[746] Emam A, Yu AR, Park HJ, Mahfoud R, Kus J, Burrows LL, and Lingwood CA. Laboratory and clinical Pseudomonas aeruginosa strains do not bind glycosphingolipids in vitro or

during type IV pili-mediated initial host cell attachment. *Microbiology* 152: pp. 2789–99, 2006.

[747] Engel J, and Eran Y. Subversion of mucosal barrier polarity by Pseudomonas aeruginosa. *Front Microbiol* 2: p. 114, 2011.

[748] Lee A, Chow D, Haus B, Tseng W, Evans D, Fleiszig S, Chandy G, and Machen T. Airway epithelial tight junctions and binding and cytotoxicity of *Pseudomonas aeruginosa*. *Am J Physiol* 277: pp. L204–17, 1999.

[749] Plotkowski MC, de Bentzmann S, Pereira SH, Zahm JM, Bajolet-Laudinat O, Roger P, and Puchelle E. *Pseudomonas aeruginosa* internalization by human epithelial respiratory cells depends on cell differentiation, polarity, and junctional complex integrity. *Am J Respir Cell Mol Biol* 20: pp. 880–90, 1999.

[750] Fleiszig SM, Evans DJ, Do N, Vallas V, Shin S, and Mostov KE. Epithelial cell polarity affects susceptibility to Pseudomonas aeruginosa invasion and cytotoxicity. *Infect Immun* 65: pp. 2861–7, 1997.

[751] Pier GB, Grout M, Zaidi TS, Olsen JC, Johnson LG, Yankaskas JR, and Goldberg JB. Role of mutant CFTR in hypersusceptibility of cystic fibrosis patients to lung infections. *Science* 271: pp. 64–7, 1996.

[752] Pier GB, Grout M, and Zaidi TS. Cystic fibrosis transmembrane conductance regulator is an epithelial cell receptor for clearance of *Pseudomonas aeruginosa* from the lung. *Proc Natl Acad Sci USA* 94: pp. 12088–93, 1997.

[753] Campodonico VL, Gadjeva M, Paradis-Bleau C, Uluer A, and Pier GB. Airway epithelial control of Pseudomonas aeruginosa infection in cystic fibrosis. *Trends Mol Med* 14: pp. 120–33, 2008.

[754] Tseng J, Do J, Widdicombe JH, and Machen TE. Innate Immune Responses of Human Tracheal Epithelium to P. aeruginosa Flagellin, TNF_α and $IL1_\beta$. *Am J Physiol* 290: pp. C678–90, 2005.

[755] Garcia-Medina R, Dunne WM, Singh PK, and Brody SL. Pseudomonas aeruginosa acquires biofilm-like properties within airway epithelial cells. *Infect Immun* 73: pp. 8298–305, 2005.

[756] Meyerholz DK, Stoltz DA, Namati E, Ramachandran S, Pezzulo AA, Smith AR, Rector MV, Suter MJ, Kao S, McLennan G, Tearney GJ, Zabner J, McCray PB, Jr., and Welsh MJ. Loss of cystic fibrosis transmembrane conductance regulator function produces abnormalities in tracheal development in neonatal pigs and young children. *Am J Respir Crit Care Med* 182: pp. 1251–61, 2010.

[757] Schiller KR, Maniak PJ, and O'Grady SM. Cystic fibrosis transmembrane conductance regulator is involved in airway epithelial wound repair. *Am J Physiol* 299: pp. C912–21, 2010.

[758] Trinh NT, Bardou O, Prive A, Maille E, Adam D, Lingee S, Ferraro P, Desrosiers MY, Coraux C, and Brochiero E. Improvement of defective cystic fibrosis airway epithelial wound repair after CFTR rescue. *Eur Respir J*, 2012.

[759] Trinh NT, Prive A, Maille E, Noel J, and Brochiero E. EGF and K+ channel activity control normal and cystic fibrosis bronchial epithelia repair. *Am J Physiol* 295: pp. L866–80, 2008.

[760] Merten MD, and Figarella C. Constitutive hypersecretion and insensitivity to neurotransmitters by cystic fibrosis tracheal gland cells. *Am J Physiol* 264: pp. L98–9, 1993.

[761] Kammouni W, Naimi D, Renaud W, Bianco N, Figarella C, and Merten MD. High lysosomal activities in cystic fibrosis tracheal gland cells corrected by adenovirus-mediated CFTR gene transfer. *Biochim Biophys Acta* 1453: pp. 14–22, 1999.

[762] Baconnais S, Delavoie F, Zahm JM, Milliot M, Terryn C, Castillon N, Banchet V, Michel J, Danos O, Merten M, Chinet T, Zierold K, Bonnet N, Puchelle E, and Balossier G. Abnormal ion content, hydration and granule expansion of the secretory granules from cystic fibrosis airway glandular cells. *Exp Cell Res* 309: pp. 296–304, 2005.

[763] Howard M, Jiang X, Stolz DB, Hill WG, Johnson JA, Watkins SC, Frizzell RA, Bruton CM, Robbins PD, and Weisz OA. Forskolin-induced apical membrane insertion of virally expressed, epitope-tagged CFTR in polarized MDCK cells. *Am J Physiol* 279: pp. C375–82, 2000.

[764] Bertrand CA, and Frizzell RA. The role of regulated CFTR trafficking in epithelial secretion. *Am J Physiol* 285: pp. C1–18, 2003.

[765] Mergey M, Lemnaouar M, Veissiere D, Perricaudet M, Gruenert DC, Picard J, Capeau J, Brahimi-Horn MC, and Paul A. CFTR gene transfer corrects defective glycoconjugate secretion in human CF epithelial tracheal cells. *Am J Physiol* 269: pp. L855–64, 1995.

[766] LeSimple P, Liao J, Robert R, Gruenert DC, and Hanrahan JW. Cystic fibrosis transmembrane conductance regulator trafficking modulates the barrier function of airway epithelial cell monolayers. *J Physiol* 588: pp. 1195–209, 2010.

[767] Kelley TJ, and Drumm ML. Inducible nitric oxide synthase expression is reduced in cystic fibrosis murine and human airway epithelial cells. *J Clin Invest* 102: pp. 1200–7, 1998.

[768] Kreiselmeier NE, Kraynack NC, Corey DA, and Kelley TJ. Statin-mediated correction of STAT1 signaling and inducible nitric oxide synthase expression in cystic fibrosis epithelial cells. *Am J Physiol* 285: pp. L1286–95, 2003.

[769] Zheng S, De BP, Choudhary S, Comhair SA, Goggans T, Slee R, Williams BR, Pilewski J, Haque SJ, and Erzurum SC. Impaired innate host defense causes susceptibility to respiratory virus infections in cystic fibrosis. *Immunity* 18: pp. 619–30, 2003.

[770] Kelley TJ, Elmer HL, and Corey DA. Reduced Smad3 protein expression and altered

transforming growth factor- beta1-mediated signaling in cystic fibrosis epithelial cells. *Am J Respir Cell Mol Biol* 25: pp. 732–8, 2001.

[771] Cannon CL, Kowalski MP, Stopak KS, and Pier GB. Pseudomonas aeruginosa-induced apoptosis is defective in respiratory epithelial cells expressing mutant cystic fibrosis trans-membrane conductance regulator. *Am J Respir Cell Mol Biol* 29: pp. 188–97, 2003.

Author Biography

Jonathan Widdicombe received a B.A. in Zoology and a D. Phil. in Pharmacology from Oxford. From 1976 to 2003 he worked at the Cardiovascular Research Institute and the Department of Physiology at the University of California - San Francisco. Since 2000, he has been a Professor of Physiology and Membrane Biology at the University of California - Davis. From 1988 to 2003, he was Director of a "Specialized Center of Research" into cystic fibrosis, funded by the National Institutes of Health.